Praise for *Doctor You*

'Jeremy Howick reveals the science behind self- healing. Read this groundbreaking book!' Deepak Chopra

'Howick provides an accessible and thoughtful explanation of what it means to be healthy and how modern health care can lead us astray. An ambitious and integrative book that is perfect if you are looking to intelligently navigate the maze of modern health care.' Ty Tashiro, author of *The Science of Happily Ever After*

'A timely book on a timeless problem of how body and mind interact to affect our health and well-being. Beautifully written by an international expert in the field, it challenges old habits of thinking and promises new ways of exploring what it means to live an integrated life.' Mark Williams, author of *Mindfulness*, Professor of Clinical Psychology and former director of the Oxford Mindfulness Centre

'Jeremy Howick knows placebos and how to make it understandable to the public. He's a philosopher who understands the big picture and a researcher who understands the details that make good science.' Ted Kaptchuk

'Engaging, informative, accessible and easy to read, Doctor You will tell you all that you need to know about how the body works. Jeremy Howick will arm you with knowledge empowering you to make the right choices when it comes to your health. A must read for anyone interested in improving their health.' Virginie Chiquri, author of *Thinking Mom's Revolution*

'This fascinating book ranges over a broad range of evidence, from telling incidents, to huge comparative scientific studies with thousands of human subjects, and many things in between, all aimed at helping you lead a more healthy, vigorous, active and meaningful life. Engagingly written by an academic who can row his own boat (really!), who is as adept at yoga as he is at statistics, it is really a good read. Imagine: Science for the Beach!' Professor Dan Moerman

JEREMY HOWICK

Doctor You

Revealing the science of self-healing

CORONET

First published in Great Britain in 2017 by Coronet
An Imprint of Hodder & Stoughton
An Hachette UK company

1

Copyright © Jeremy Howick 2017

The right of Jeremy Howick to be identified as the Author of
the Work has been asserted by him in accordance with the
Copyright, Designs and Patents Act 1988.

A CIP catalogue record for this title is available from the British Library

ISBN 9781473654204
eBook ISBN 9781473654235
Tradeback ISBN 9781473654211

Typeset in Bembo MT by Palimpsest Book Production Ltd, Falkirk, Stirlingshire

Printed and bound in Great Britain by Clays Ltd, St Ives plc

Hodder & Stoughton policy is to use papers that are natural, renewable
and recyclable products and made from wood grown in sustainable forests.
The logging and manufacturing processes are expected to conform to the
environmental regulations of the country of origin.

For Mom

. . . to most medical people, this way of thinking simply makes no sense at all; rather, it makes as much sense as filling up the gas tank with Earl Grey tea.

David Morris, American writer
and interdisciplinary researcher

Does this mean that we might double our gas mileage if we wished for it hard enough? Well, no. But people are not machines, and we shouldn't treat them as such.

Dan Moerman, American medical
anthropologist

Contents

Preface

Rowing is a sport for dreamers
As long as you put in the work, you can own the dream
When the work stops, the dream disappears
> Jim Dietz, American Olympic rower
> (1972, 1976, 1980) and Olympic team coach

There were a lot of great things about my brief stint rowing for Canada in the 1990s. After spending the fall, winter and spring pushing my mental and physical limits, summer was racing season. I travelled to races with amazing teammates all over Canada and the US, as well as to the UK, France, Italy, Spain, Poland, Chile and Zambia. When things went well, we ended up standing on the podium for national or international championship medals. Then occasionally a less fun thing would happen: some of us were escorted off the podium to test for drugs. I liked the idea of drug testing as I did not want to race against cheats. But being taken away from the podium put a damper on the celebration. And the test was embarrassing, because it involved someone watching you pee in a bottle.

The testing also made you paranoid when you got ill and had to take medicine, because some athletes said that taking a routine medication made them test positive for banned drugs. I was pretty sure they were telling the truth sometimes, but I could not be sure. So, when I developed an allergy to a cat that my mother bought when I was living at home one winter, I was worried at the prospect of having to take medication. Yet I had to do something, because my nose was running, I was sneezing, and I could not sleep well. The lack of sleep made it impossible to train properly. My performance began to suffer.

I visited the allergy doctor, who pricked my skin about thirty times with different allergens to see which one made my skin turn red. He found that I was allergic to cats, dogs and dust, and prescribed a nasal spray. I looked carefully at its ingredients, and stopped at the word 'corticosteroid'. Were corticosteroids the same thing as steroids that are banned substances, I wondered? I decided not to use the spray until I found out.

I wrote to Sports Canada in Ottawa to ask whether the nasal spray was banned; however, weeks went by and I still had not received a reply. Part of the reason that officials at Sports Canada may take their time in replying to such requests could be if they believe that most people who contact them with such questions are trying to figure out ways to game the system. So I was stuck: I could not sleep or train properly, but I could not take the meds that would make me better. As a last resort, I accepted my mother's suggestion to meet her friend who was a herbal doctor. I was sceptical, but I had nothing to lose, so I made an appointment.

I visited the herbal doctor in her office not far from where I lived. She offered me a seat on her sofa, which I accepted. I had expected rows of shelves laden with jars of herbal remedies and crystals, but there were none. On the contrary, it seemed like a regular doctor's office, only calmer and cleaner. She was very professional. She took an interest in my allergies as well as other things going on in my life. We talked about my symptoms, the stress of being ill, and the hyper-competitiveness of top-level rowing. After an hour of talking, I felt very calm and she gave me her prescription. She told me to keep my head and neck warm, and to drink ginger tea twice per day.

I did not believe her treatment would work, but figured wearing a scarf and woolly hat was generally a good thing during winter in Canada, and ginger tea would not kill me. I gave it a try. After one day of drinking the ginger tea, I was surprised that I felt a bit better. After three days, I stopped sneezing almost completely, I slept well, and my nose almost stopped running altogether.

The fact that the tea seemed to work got my inherently inquisitive mind racing. (I was that annoying kid who asks their teachers and parents 'Why?' all the time.) Could my allergies have disappeared spontaneously? Or did ginger tea work because I believed it might – in other words, had it acted as a placebo? If it was 'just' a placebo effect (basically: the effect of my belief, more about that in Chapter Four), did that matter if it helped? How did my body heal itself? Had the calming effect of the herbal doctor taking time to listen to me talk made the difference? On top of all that, were there any financial barriers to selling ginger tea as an allergy cure? After all, you can't patent ginger tea, so no company can afford to spend money researching or marketing it. Searching for answers to these questions ignited a fascination that has shaped my life ever since.

Looking back, I can see that my visit to the herbal doctor was one of those pivotal moments in life that seem unimportant at the time, but in fact lead to important changes in direction. My undergraduate degree was in engineering and I had planned to become an investment banker. I dropped that idea and moved to the UK to do a PhD with leading philosophers of medicine at the London School of Economics. The philosophy provided me with a theoretical understanding of placebos and the complex ethical questions around them. I then got a job at Oxford, where I trained as a clinical epidemiologist (which is a geek word for someone who uses statistical techniques to find out whether treatments work).

I have now done ten years of research in this area, during which time I have published almost one hundred scholarly articles and a textbook. I have found answers to many of my questions. I've always been inspired by teaching and coaching others, so naturally I wanted to share what I learned. Unfortunately, the science I present in this book – a lot of which I have been involved with – has generally until now

3

been restricted to academic journals that are written in a way that nobody outside a small field reads or understands. When it is picked up outside academia, it is often by journalists who are great communicators, but who often exaggerate. The headline 'New drug to cure all forms of cancer' is much sexier than 'New drug might reduce the risk of cancer in some mice'. Most medical advances, including the ones I describe in this book, are real and important, yet are more modest than headlines frequently mislead you to believe.

Because the hard science of self-healing has rarely been shared in an understandable and accurate way, I felt compelled to write this book. I've tried to communicate the methods and results of the scientific studies in a way that is at once accurate, entertaining, and memorable. This was not easy, since as anyone who has done it knows, real science is messy, and all studies have flaws (I explain many of these in Chapter Two). Translating this complex science into a language most people can understand was like walking a tightrope in a storm. As with any writing, a serious sceptic could criticize the way I have interpreted and explained things. In spite of this, I'm confident that the main conclusions I draw in the book are correct. To anyone interested in checking the facts, I've included hundreds of references to support all the claims I make. I kept the references out of the body of the book and placed them at the end to improve readability.

Beyond doing and writing about the research, I've lived by it. Inspired by ancient philosophers and scientists who used what they learned to lead better lives, I've used my research to guide me. For example, I've refused knee and back surgery even when doctors have strongly recommended it, I avoid medicine unless it is absolutely necessary, and I've done all the exercises that are at the end of the chapters. I've also won two professional Muay Thai fights in Thailand as a (crazy?) experiment to overcome fear, I got a black belt in Tai Kwon Do to see how flexible I could be, I have done long fasts and silent meditation retreats to see how much I could calm my mind, and I became a highly qualified yoga teacher. None of this means that I've achieved perfect mental or physical health. I haven't. In fact, and as you'll see in the book, one of my motivations for becoming interested in health is that I was – and still can be – too anxious. So using the research to inform how I live just means that I can explain the geeky science by drawing on my own experience, and that I'm only recommending to others things that I'm doing or have done myself. Basically I'm swallowing my own medicine, and I like it.

This brings us to you. By the time you reach the end of the book, I hope you will have gained the things from reading it that I gained from researching and writing it. I hope you embody what you learn to actually experience better health and to help others achieve better health (as you'll see in Chapters Eleven and Twelve, your health is connected to the health of those around you). I help you achieve this by providing takeaway exercises at the end of each chapter. But don't be misled: this is not a standard self-help book; it is both less and much more. It is less, because I have not given you a quick-fix formula to help you lose seven pounds in seven days, an app that will enlighten you in a minute, or a miracle cure for late-stage cancer. I do not tell you about a trick that will make you a billion dollars or get a Hollywood star body.

On the other hand, it is much more than a standard self-help book, because it aims to change how we think about medicine and our bodies. The exercises prompt you to experience that your body is an extraordinary entity whose different parts are capable of compensating, healing and regenerating themselves much more often than you may believe. The exercises are a way for you to become the protagonist of *Doctor You*, the subject of your own experiment. The new way of thinking that the book encourages will guide you in many more ways that I can list in a single book and that are personal to you.

Here are just a few examples. If you knew that your body produced its own morphine, would you take as much aspirin – which can make your stomach bleed – for mild headaches? If you knew getting together with a friend had the same biological effect on depression as a pill, would you be less likely to try Prozac – which can have side effects ranging from sexual dysfunction to suicidal tendencies? If you knew that placebo knee surgery was as good as the real thing, would you choose the surgeon's knife before trying physiotherapy? Your answers to these questions will evolve as you read the book – either by changing your mind or by making you more confident that you made the correct choice in the first place. You will learn enough about medical evidence to arrive at good answers to your health questions alongside healthcare professionals. You will no longer be at the constant mercy of (admittedly sometimes wonderful) drugs, devices and surgery that has become overused.

Most importantly, I hope you enjoy reading this book as much as I enjoyed writing it.

Introduction

Too Much Medicine

The body is the house of God
            proverb of the External Temple of Luxor, Egypt

In the last century we have discovered antibiotics to cure deadly infections, surgical techniques to transplant hearts, and cures for most forms of infertility. Many of us alive today would have long since died were it not for some of the astonishing medical advances seen in recent decades. We live an average of twenty years longer than our great-grandparents. Calling modern medicine a scientific miracle is no exaggeration. That is why I have used it, you have used it, and we should all be grateful that we can continue using it. We will also benefit from, and should therefore encourage, more medical research.

Yet even as the best individual drugs have some bad side effects, modern medicine as a whole has some unintended and harmful consequences. We are using too much of it, it can be risky, it is bankrupting us, and we have forgotten how remarkable our own bodies are at healing without medicine.

One in seven boys in the US are diagnosed with ADHD if they can't sit still in school. One in ten adults in developed nations take antidepressant drugs that have harmful side effects and can lead to dependence. Statins are recommended for everyone over forty as a way to lower cholesterol in the blood, yet there is a debate about whether they work at all for people with low baseline risks. Some elderly (over sixty-five years old) people get antipsychotic drugs to prevent

7

dementia, although most will never experience it. More than half of elderly Americans, British and Canadians take at least five prescription drugs each day, with some taking over twenty, their lives a non-stop ritual of pill popping then managing side effects.

All of this can be deadly. Prescription painkillers kill more people than heroin and cocaine combined in the US, overuse of antibiotics is creating dangerous superbugs, and eighty per cent of people who take several pills at a time have side effects ranging from shortness of breath to death. In fact, medical errors are the third leading cause of death in the US, just behind cancer and respiratory disease. Fatal prescription-drug errors alone kill over 100,000 people each year in the US.

We all want treatments to help out-of-control young boys, but it is hard to believe that one in seven of them need meth-amphetamines to survive going to school. Most people would want the option of taking antidepressant drugs for serious depression, but do ten per cent of people in the developed world really need them? And of course we want our elderly friends and family to remain mentally alert, but it is hard to believe that they all need to be given potentially dangerous antipsychotics to prevent dementia that may never appear. In fact, recent research is starting to show that when elderly people *stop* taking some of their prescription drugs, they fare better than those who carry on taking all of them.

The overuse of medicine is not only unhealthy: it is in danger of bankrupting us. Americans spend over 300 billion dollars on prescription drugs every year, Canadians spend over 28 billion, and medical costs in the UK have almost doubled (in real terms) in the last decade.

Because of all this unnecessary treatment, expense and harm, it is tempting to reject modern medicine altogether, and that is just what some people do. Conspiracy theories about corrupt Big Pharma abound, with some claiming that all drugs are bad. This view is grounded in some valid facts. Glaring financial conflicts of interest guide the research agenda to areas that are profitable for the companies, but not necessarily health priorities.

Worse, some pharmaceutical companies have been shown to manipulate their results to make their drugs look more effective and less harmful than they actually are. They also sometimes take fairly normal mental traits, give them new names, and classify them as diseases so that they can sell pills they happen to have manufactured to solve these 'problems'. For example, most of us have trouble focusing on things sometimes – it is normal. Yet there is now a name for it: adult attention deficit disorder, which can be treated by methamphetamines (speed). There is an increasing worry that diseases are being exaggerated and even invented to sell cures – this is called 'disease mongering'. All this needs to change by aligning the interests of our health with those of profit.

But rejecting all pharmaceutical drugs goes too far. Many drugs work: morphine reduces pain, adrenaline successfully treats anaphylactic shock, statins prevent heart disease in high-risk individuals, and polio vaccines prevent polio, to name just a few. The problem arises when we let pharmaceutical companies evaluate their own products. If we let them get away with this, we should not blame them for coming up with results that suit their interests. The answer to the conflict-of-interest problem is to campaign for the independent and transparent evaluation of drugs.

This is starting to happen, perhaps most notably due to Ben Goldacre and his growing team of researchers at Oxford. We also need business for innovation, because academics are simply too slow (trust me). Finally, there are actually some good pharmaceutical companies out there, with the Mario Negri Institute in Milan leading the way. Following Jonas Salk, who refused to patent the polio vaccine – he famously said, 'You can't patent the sun' – Mario Negri refuses to patent their discoveries in order to make their drugs affordable to all. These stories are just a few showing it is not true that all drug companies are evil.

Another way people reject modern medicine is by becoming too trusting of alternatives. Some forms of alternative medicine, especially acupuncture for back pain, are now scientifically proven to be effective and are safer than many more 'conventional' options such as surgery. Alternative practitioners are also often better at exploiting placebo effects, and the benefits of mind/body self-healing, much more effectively than conventional medicine.

But it is not true that all alternative treatments benefit people, and there is rarely proof that they work better than conventional options. Also, the alternative medicine industry is exactly that: an industry. As such, they fall prey to the same conflict of interest problems as pharmaceutical companies, albeit on a much smaller scale because there is less money in it. Finally, many alternative healers often ask patients to accept a spiritual worldview that some find hard to swallow.

The good news is that there is a middle way that neither condemns all pharmaceutical drugs nor praises all alternatives. The middle way transcends that dichotomy and uses modern medicine's *method* (mega-studies called 'systematic reviews' and more about these in the next chapter) to investigate mind-body self-healing. I have spent the last ten years doing these systematic reviews. I will go into much more detail about these reviews in the upcoming pages, but here is a summary:

- My review with over 15,000 patients found that placebo treatments have the same-sized effects as 'real' treatments.
- My review with almost 1,500 patients showed that doctors who give positive messages to patients can reduce pain by as much as aspirin and other over-the-counter drugs.
- My review with over 5,000 patients found that when doctors are empathic and offer hopeful messages, patient pain, satisfaction and ability to function (such as walk upstairs), go up, while pain, anxiety, depression, irritable

bowel syndrome (IBS) symptoms and asthma symptoms are reduced by between ten and twenty per cent. Positive thoughts can influence 'physical' outcomes such as the amount of medication patients take, the speed of hand movement in Parkinson's patients, and lung activity. Unfortunately, the evidence in this area is not being implemented, partly because many doctors are overloaded with paperwork.

- In another one of my studies, I identified sixty-four studies with approximately 5,000 patients. I found that while some practitioners are very good at communicating hope and empathy, many are not. Male healthcare practitioners were less empathetic than female practitioners, and practitioners in Australia, the US and the UK were considered to be more empathetic than their colleagues in Germany and China.
- My review of open-label placebos (placebos that patients *know* are placebos – I solve the mystery of how these work in Chapter Nine) included 260 patients who had either IBS, depression, allergic rhinitis, back pain or attention deficit hyperactivity disorder (ADHD). The effects were positive for all the trials.
- My survey showed that ninety-seven per cent of UK doctors have prescribed a placebo at least once in their career.

Other researchers have also conducted systematic reviews in this area and have shown that relaxation and meditation can reduce symptoms of asthma, anxiety, heart disease, depression, insomnia, diabetes, back pain and stress, and increase a sense of wellbeing. A systematic review with fifty-three trials showed that placebo surgery was as good as 'real' surgery more than half of the time. Another systematic review with over 300,000 people found that people who had closer connections to family and friends lived longer than those who did not, and that being socially isolated is as bad for health as smoking. Positive thinking, empathy and placebos can no longer be viewed as fuzzy things that affect 'soft' outcomes: there is even evidence that they affect your brain and your DNA.

The problems with too much medicine, combined with the growing science of mind/body medicine, have reached a tipping point, and people are taking notice. For example, in October 2016 the telegenic Dr Chris van Tulleken presented a BBC television show called *The Doctor Who Gave Up Drugs*. Chris met patients who were taking pills for depression or pain and told them, 'I can do anything for you . . . except give you pills.'

In one instance, a woman called Sarah had been on anti-depressants for eight years and could not get off them. Chris made her swim in an ice-cold lake (among other things) and she was able to stop taking pills. Another woman called Wendy had chronic shoulder pain for twenty years. Chris replaced her drugs with placebo pills and made her do daily exercises and her pain went away. Watching this show confirmed that I was not alone in thinking that there is another way for medicine. The evidence for mind/body self-healing points us in a direction that can make us happier, healthier, and save us a lot of money.

PART I

Evidence of Self-Healing
(and How You Know)

Take care of your body. It's the only place you have to live
Jim Rohn, American entrepreneur,
author and motivational speaker

. . . it is not necessary for us to understand all the technical
details in order to understand what is going on in the world
and exercise what I call an 'active economic citizenship' to
demand the right courses of action to those in decision-
making positions
Ha-Joon Chang,
Professor of Economics at Cambridge University

If all the medicine we use today was necessary, the human race would not have survived long enough to discover it. Before modern medicine, many humans lived until they were over eighty years old, the Inuit survived without electricity in the incredibly harsh arctic climate, and Vikings rowed from Denmark to Newfoundland. Without any medicine, your body takes care of most infections, heals most broken bones, and gets rid of most depressive episodes. Our body makes its own morphine, growth hormones and pleasure drug (dopamine). It even has a kind of cell whose scientific name is 'natural killer', which can fight unwanted viruses and tumours. That is why it should not surprise you that my study showed placebo effects are often as large as treatment effects, and my survey showed that most doctors use them.

Sceptics reading this have already asked *how do we know* any of this? That is a good question, because we are bombarded every day with claims about a new diet, exercise fads, and promises of new, magic-bullet cancer drugs. These treatments all need to be evaluated rigorously and scientifically in what I will call 'fair tests'. The basics of fair tests are not that hard to grasp. If you understand what a fair race is, you can understand what a rigorous scientific test is. Basically, you can think of a fair race as a test of a new treatment compared with a placebo. If the new treatment is proven to be consistently better than a placebo, then we can say it works, and if a placebo consistently outperforms doing nothing, then the placebo works.

But first let me tell you a few things about your body that might surprise you.

I

Your Amazing Body

. . . if a cold is treated energetically it will get well in seven days, while if left to itself it will get well in a week . . .
Royal Navy Commander W. A. Hopkins

How 20,000 prisoners of war survived on 600 calories a day

Archie Cochrane was the esteemed Scottish medical doctor who died in 1988. He inspired the creation of the Cochrane Collaboration, which is an international organisation that organises medical research systematically and produces what many believe is the most trusted source of evidence. He was a also doctor in a prisoner-of-war (POW) camp during the Second World War. He wrote about one of his experiences here:

> I was usually the senior medical officer and for a considerable time the only officer and the only doctor. (It was bad enough being a POW, but having me as your doctor was a bit too much.) There were about 20,000 POWs in the camp, of whom a quarter were British. The diet was about 600 calories a day and we all had diarrhoea. In addition we had severe epidemics of typhoid, diphtheria, infections, jaundice, and sand-fly fever, with more than 300 cases of 'pitting oedema above the knee'. To cope with this, we had a ramshackle hospital, some aspirin, some antacid, and some skin antiseptic.
>
> The only real assets were some devoted orderlies, mainly from the Friends' Field Ambulance Unit. Under the best conditions one would have expected an appreciable mortality; there in the Dulag I expected hundreds to die of diphtheria alone in the absence of specific therapy. In point of fact there were only four deaths, of which three were due to gunshot wounds inflicted by the Germans. This excellent result had,

of course, nothing to do with the therapy they received or my clinical skill. It demonstrated, on the other hand, very clearly the relative unimportance of therapy in comparison with the recuperative power of the human body. On one occasion, when I was the only doctor there, I asked the German Stabsarzt for more doctors to help me cope with these fantastic problems. He replied: 'Nein! Aerzte sind ueber-fluessig.' ('No! Doctors are superfluous.') I was furious and even wrote a poem about it; later I wondered if he was wise or cruel; he was certainly right.

Of course, most POWs are not average people. The soldiers in Cochrane's story were young and – at least before they were captured – healthier than most people. If the camp had been full of older and sick prisoners, there almost certainly would have been more deaths. This is what medical geeks like me call 'selection bias', because healthy people were 'selected' to be soldiers in the first place. Still, the poor living conditions and rampant disease-epidemics are bad for young healthy people, too, and even a good doctor like Cochrane expected many more deaths. Cochrane's story shows us how amazing human bodies actually are. It is a funny thing that some of the most fascinating facts about the human body are not taught (or at least not taught in a way that students remember them) in medical school.

Ten things you probably didn't know about your body that might blow your mind

Here are a few facts about your body:

- Pound for pound, your bones are stronger than steel, since a bar of steel of comparable size would weigh several times more. In principle (if you could prevent it from buckling – for example, by taking a piece of it), a human thigh bone can support 19,000 pounds (8,500 kilograms), which is as much as five pickup trucks.

- Your stomach acid is strong enough to melt zinc.
- You have about thirty trillion cells in your body, and each one of them is alive. Thirty trillion is such a big number that it is almost impossible for the human brain to fathom how awesome it is. It is thirty times a thousand times a thousand times a million. You would have to live 63,000 years to be just *one* trillion seconds old.
- The adult human brain has 100 billion neurons with close to a thousand trillion connections between them. Each neuron makes between 1,000 and 10,000 connections with other neurons in the brain. This means that the number of combinations of brain-relationship activity is more than the number of elementary particles in the known universe.
- On average, your body is just ten years old. Your skin completely regenerates every seven days. Your liver completely regenerates itself every year or so. It has been estimated that the average cell in your body is between seven and ten years old at most. So no matter how many years have passed between now and when you were born, your body is less than ten years old, on average. The only parts of your body that last a lifetime seem to be your brain, heart muscles, and the inner-lens cells of the eye. However, recent research shows that some brain cells (the ganglia cells) do in fact renew themselves.
- During the process of regeneration your body produces cells with mutant DNA that could become cancerous if they divided. However, in normal circumstances a powerful protein called P-53 stops cancer dead in its tracks by activating repairs to damaged DNA or killing off cells that are beyond repair.
- If all the blood cells in your body were lined up end-to-end, they would be 100,000 kilometres long. This is enough to wrap around the earth more than twice.
- Your lymphatic system, which is responsible for removing body toxins, is much less known, but contains about twice as many kilometres of vessels as the blood circulation

system. Laid end-to-end, the lymphatic vessels would wrap around the earth more than five times.

- Your heart beats one hundred thousand times per day, and over three billion times in an average lifetime. During this time, most hearts never need a repair or check-up.
- Nerve signals from your brain travel up to 170 miles (270 kilometres) per hour.

Your immune system deserves a closer look.

The scientific name for natural killer cells is natural killer cells

You cannot avoid the fact that millions of germs, viruses, toxins and parasites enter your body every day, many of which want to attack you. When you breathe, they come into your nose, mouth, throat and lungs. When you eat they come into your stomach. And when you get a scratch, they get into your bloodstream. Without an immune system, some of these invaders would literally eat your flesh to the bone in a couple of weeks. That is why corpses – which do not have immune systems to protect them – are actually eaten by parasites. Your immune system deals with these millions of daily invaders silently and effortlessly without you even being aware.

Your skin acts as a first line of defence against foreign invaders. Skin has lots of disease-fighting, white blood cells in case you get a scratch. When you inhale harmful viruses and germs, mucus in your nose and throat also acts as a defence. The mucus in your throat takes in unwanted particles. Once absorbed, they are swallowed into the stomach, where your stomach acid kills them quickly.

In the unlikely event that some stubborn bacteria or virus gets past the mucus in your throat to your lungs, the lungs meet them with their own specially designed immune system. The microenvironment of the alveoli (tiny air sacs that make up the lungs) is very delicate and would be damaged if the immune system were constantly on high alert there. So the specially adapted immune system in the lungs remains in a steady-state mode, and kicks into full-on attack-mode only when germs are present.

If disease-causing germs get past the mucus in your throat to your stomach, the gastric acid down there will take care of them. Gastric acid is strong enough to kill most harmful bacteria that might get that far. Amazingly, the acid does not destroy the elements we require for our own nourishment like sugar and fat, and it even helps digest protein. In some rare cases, potentially harmful bacteria or viruses manage to get through the stomach to the intestine, sometimes hidden within a piece of food. If that happens, helpful bacteria within the intestine usually eliminate them.

If some harmful germ escapes the mucus in the throat, the acid in the stomach, and the good bacteria in your intestine and makes it into the bloodstream, another line of defence gets activated. The heroes of the part of the immune system in the blood are the white blood cells, which I have already mentioned. There are different types of white blood cells and they are everywhere, about half a million per drop of blood. The number increases when you get an infection.

Big white blood cells called macrophages engulf invaders whole and essentially starve them to death, then digest them. If some germs escape the macrophage, another kind of white blood cell seeks out and kills the infected cells. These highly trained killers specialise in 'seeking and destroying' any cells that have been compromised. A common type of white blood cells that do seek and destroy missions are called natural killer cells. The first time I heard the name 'natural killer cell' I thought it was a nickname to explain these cells to people who are learning about the immune system. It is not: 'natural killer cell' is the real name. Your immune system even has a memory, so that the second time invaders come, it can mount their attack more quickly. This is why people only get some diseases like chickenpox once.

Your inner pharmacy

Besides protecting you from invaders, your body has an inner pharmacy that can reduce pain, combat depression, and generally make you feel good. Your body produces its own *endorphins*, which create the natural high that people report when running or doing yoga. Endorphins derive their name from two other words: *endogenous*, which means 'produced within a system' (in your body), and *morphine*. Squish the words '*endo*genous' and 'mo*rphine*' together and you get endorphin. An endorphin is morphine produced inside your body. Really. Morphine and endorphin molecules are almost identical, and from the point of view of the body, they are identical. The same substance that some drug addicts are addicted to, or that doctors give to people in severe pain, is produced right inside your body.

Your inner drug factory also produces other drugs. It makes growth hormones that help cells reproduce and regenerate (it is also the same thing that is illegal for athletes to inject), dopamine that makes you feel good (and has the same effect as taking cocaine), and many other powerful chemicals. I will tell you a lot more about this in Part III.

Three questions that you may have

I will finish this chapter by answering three questions that many people have when I tell them how amazing their bodies are.

If the body can heal itself, is it our fault if we get ill?

NO. We are all born with different bodies – different genetic makeups – and different environments. We have different tendencies to think certain ways. I was born in Canada, which is a rich country, where my mother was a fantastic cook who instilled healthy eating habits and my father insisted on exercise, hard work and high standards. And mostly I have been blessed with great loyal friends. I had little control over those things, and they gave me some healthy habits and a good social network.

At the same time the high expectations placed on me made me feel anxious sometimes. I did not have much control of that either. Just as I didn't have control over most of my background, you did not have control over yours. And even if you did have control over something you did, blaming anything or anyone – including yourself – will not change it. In fact, blame is likely to increase your stress and make you less healthy. What matters is that your body *is* amazing and, no matter what your current health status is, chances are you can improve it, even if only a little bit. (The one slight caveat to this answer is people with very serious or terminal illnesses. Yet even in these cases the right attitude can bring peace and happiness, and I talk about this in Chapter Ten.)

If our bodies are so amazing, why do we die or get ill?

Despite all the wonderful discoveries that science has made, there are a lot of mysteries we have not cracked, including the details of the ageing process. Unless you have 'Syndrome X' (a real but rare disease that prevents people from ageing) you will age and eventually die, because you are mortal. Considering how many bacteria and germs we eat, how much stress we put our bodies under, and how much junk we consume, it is actually pretty surprising that we are not a lot more ill than we are.

If our bodies are so amazing, why do we need medicine?

Usually you do not need medicine. Many of the 'illnesses' that most of us get – things like back pain, mild depression, anxiety, ADHD and minor injuries – go away without medicine.

The fact that we often take medicine and then we feel better may lead us to believe that medication is necessary whenever we are sick. But the truth is that much of the time our bodies would have healed themselves even without drugs. For in most cases our cold will go away whether or not we take vitamin C, our headaches will go away whether or not we take aspirin, and our mild depression will go away whether or not we take Prozac. If we want to know whether a medication is truly effective, we have to look at the evidence, which is the topic of the next two chapters.

Takeaway: Take the brake off negative stuff – in fact, throw it into the garbage

Most of us do not realise how amazing our bodies are. In fact, we have too many negative thoughts. Cognitive behavioural therapists say there is something called our 'inner critic', which automatically interprets things in a negative way. Here are seven common types of negative thoughts that we often have:

1. *All or nothing thinking, with no grey areas*: 'I can't follow this exercise programme/diet/lifestyle,' or 'I tried to make a change before and it didn't work, so nothing will ever work, there's no point.'
2. *Crystal-ball gazing and mind-reading other people*: 'They must think I look stupid,' or 'People must think I am unattractive,' or 'There's no point in trying to make myself healthier. It won't work.'
3. *Disqualifying the positive*: 'I may be pretty good at cooking healthy food, but anybody can do that.'
4. *Drama queen*: 'I can't find my purse. I'm losing my memory.'
5. *Unrealistic expectations*: 'I should keep going, even when I'm exhausted.'

24

6. *Name calling, to self and others*: 'Silly fool,' or 'If people really knew me, they wouldn't like me.'
7. *Catastrophising*: 'Nothing is ever going to work for me.'

The vast majority are false, and even fewer are helpful. They are also a common cause of many mental-health disorders, so it is good to reduce them as much as we can. Cognitive behavioural therapy (CBT) helps people use new thought-patterns so that negative thoughts stop having a bad effect on how people feel and behave. There are many trials showing that CBT can help cure people who are depressed, anxious and low in self-esteem, in large part by helping them transcend negative thought-patterns.

I am not a CBT therapist, but a CBT therapist taught me a very easy technique that often works very well. And it works quickly. I was complaining about some negative thought I was having. I think it was that I wasn't feeling happy in spite of some recent achievements. His advice was:

Imagine that you are walking on the street and there are some mischievous small children running around who are no taller than your waist. Imagine one of them tries to steal your wallet from your back pocket. What would you do? You wouldn't get upset, you would simply brush their hands away from your back pocket gently, yet very firmly and positively. Then you would forget it and carry on your journey. You can do the same thing with thoughts. If any negative thoughts arise that you don't like, imagine you are brushing them away firmly the same way you would brush away a child's hand from your wallet.

The next time a negative thought arises, realise it is probably not true and brush it away. Move on with your life to things that make you feel better. (Note to anyone not interested in how we get good evidence: skip the next two chapters and move straight to Chapter Four.)

2

When to Trust the Evidence

A doctor and a lawyer were talking at a party, but they weren't having fun because people kept interrupting to tell the doctor about their health problems and ask for free medical advice. After a while, the annoyed doctor asked the lawyer, 'How do you stop people from asking you for legal advice when you're at a party?'

'I give it to them,' replied the lawyer, 'then I send them a bill.'

The doctor was shocked, but agreed to give it a try. The next day, still feeling slightly guilty, he prepared the bills for the people who had asked him for advice the previous night. When he went to place them in his mailbox, he found a bill from the lawyer.

I am not a medical doctor, but as a medical researcher people ask me the same kinds of questions they might ask their doctor at a party. What do I think about herbal medicine? Do the benefits of chemotherapy outweigh the side effects? Can medical marijuana cure depression? What about vaccines and autism? The answer to these questions can only be found by looking at the *evidence*. If there is good evidence a treatment works, we can probably trust it; otherwise we should be careful. We will probably all need to know whether a particular treatment works at some point, so we should all understand what good evidence is. The problem is that the media love splashing headlines about 'magic bullet' treatments before there is evidence proving they work and, with very few exceptions, academics use incomprehensible mumbo-jumbo to explain their studies. Worse, academics rarely bother to translate their research for other researchers, let alone members of the lay public. So someone with a PhD in chemistry will have difficulty understanding what someone with a PhD in physics writes.

Yet if you want to get the basics, evidence is easy to understand, as long as it is explained clearly. I translated the language of medical researchers for my philosophy colleagues in my book *The Philosophy of Evidence-Based Medicine*, and in this chapter I'm translating it for you. What you'll find is that for most things you do not need to understand more than the basics and that is enough to become an 'active medical citizen'.

A fair start and randomised trials

I could tell everyone that I ran one hundred metres faster than Usain Bolt. But nobody would believe me unless I proved it by lining up beside him, racing, and winning. If I refused to race him, you would say I was full of s**t. Yet that kind of bulls**t is common in medicine. To prove a treatment works, you have to compare it with what happens if someone does not take the treatment – you have to have a 'race'.

For example, a researcher, often one who was paid by industry, might give you vitamin C when you caught a cold. Then, if your cold went away in five days, he might say the cold had gone because of the vitamin C. But most colds go away in five days without any treatment anyway. To check whether taking vitamin C helps, you need to compare people who take it with people who don't. Only if the colds in the group that got vitamin C went away faster than the other group could we say that vitamin C 'won'. But the start of the race would have to be fair . . .

If I agreed to prove myself by actually racing Usain Bolt, but then took a massive head-start, you would say the race was not fair. While it is not always on purpose, this kind of cheating is common in medical research. For instance, a researcher might give younger, healthier people vitamin C and not give vitamin C to older, less healthy people. But since young and healthy people's colds go away faster than older, unhealthy people's colds, that would not prove anything, because they had a 'head start' when it comes to health.

The groups that take or do not take vitamin C have to be as similar as possible. To create similar groups, scientists flip a coin to decide who gets vitamin C and who does not. (Actually, they don't really flip a coin, but they use a computer to achieve the same thing.) When we flip a coin to decide who gets what, we have a fair start and what is called a randomised trial.

Blinding to stop cheating along the way

At the 2016 cycling world championships, a Belgian cyclist was caught with a hidden motor in their bicycle. (The cyclist claimed it was not their bike, and that the team mechanic had given them the wrong bike by accident.) Whether or not they knew, having the motor was cheating. Yet this kind of cheating is also common in medical research, although it is not always done on purpose. If the doctor believes vitamin C works (or if they are being paid by the company who makes a drug to do the test), then they might interpret a little sniffle as failure to cure the person who did not take vitamin C, but as a cure for the person who took the vitamin C. The same goes for the patients and everyone else involved in the trial. If people believe that the treatment works, they can make biased observations, or pretend to get better when in fact they don't. The coolest study I know that shows this is called 'Pygmalion in the Classroom'.

In the spring of 1964, Robert Rosenthal and Lenore Jacobsen went to a public (meaning state-funded in the US) elementary school called the 'Oak School' (the real name is withheld) to carry out an experiment, which they named after Pygmalion, the Greek artist who sculpted an ivory statue that came to life because he lavished it with so much attention.

28

Rosenthal and Jacobsen gave all five hundred kids in grades 1–5 (kids between five and ten years old) a test they called the impressive-sounding 'Harvard Test of Inflected Acquisition'. Teachers were told that the test 'predicts the likelihood that a child will show a learning spurt within the near future'. Teachers administered the multiple-choice test, and two independent assessors, who did not know the identities of the participants, scored them separately. The teachers were allowed to see the results of both tests, but were told not to discuss them with the pupils or their parents. After a year, the same Harvard test was administered by the teachers and graded by the same independent assessors. The students that Rosenthal and Jacobsen had originally scored as in the top twenty per cent for learning-spurt potential improved in English, Maths, and even IQ, significantly more than the other students.

The funny thing was: the Harvard Text of Inflected Acquisition was actually a standard IQ test. Then, Rosenthal and Jacobsen did not choose the *top* twenty per cent of students, they chose twenty per cent at random! The reason these students 'spurted' was not because they were 'spurters', but because the teachers believed in them. A teacher, believing that a student was ready to 'spurt', might pay special attention to that student. The additional attention received could easily translate into accelerated rates of improvement.

Pygmalion-type effects are probably common in medical research. When a doctor or researcher believes they are administering the best experimental treatment to a patient, they might treat that group differently than they would a patient who was getting the placebo instead of the experimental treatment. Meanwhile, if the doctor believed that a different patient was being given a placebo, the doctor might not bother providing the highest quality of care. They might deem it 'not worthwhile', especially given that they all have limited time to distribute among their many patients. An obvious scenario where caregiver knowledge could have an effect is when they have a personal or financial interest in showing that the experimental treatment works. The role of these personal or financial interests can be conscious or unconscious.

To prevent bias, researchers are 'blinded', which means they do not know which patients get the experimental treatment. To achieve blinding, you obviously need to give some patients placebos that can be disguised as a drug. This is possible with pills, but much more difficult with complicated treatments like ginger tea and exercise.

In practice, blinding is not easy to achieve because researchers can be very good at figuring out which patients got the real treatment. The way researchers hide their knowledge of which patients get the real drug and which patients get the placebo is that they have a secret number for each patient. For instance, one patient might be assigned the number '2958' and another will be given the number '5829'. Then, in a separate place, the 'decoding' for the numbers is done. This can be a piece of paper saying '2958 = placebo' and '5829 = drug'.

Sometimes researchers and doctors can try to decode the numbers themselves. Kenneth Schulz is a prolific researcher who is the president of the Quantitative Sciences Department within the International Clinical Studies Support Center. He conducted a workshop where investigators revealed anonymously the methods they used to figure out which patient was getting which treatment. Here is what he reported about one of them:

> Still another workshop participant had attempted to decipher a numbered container scheme, but had given up after her attempts bore no success. One evening she noticed a light on in the principal investigator's office and dropped in to say hello. Instead of finding the principal investigator, she found an attending physician who also was involved in the same trial. He unabashedly announced that he was rifling the files for the assignment sequence, because he had not

been able to decipher it any other way. What materialized was almost as curious as her response. She admitted being impressed with his diligence and proceeded to help in rifling the files.

The Pygmalion experiment shows that when a doctor believes they are giving the best treatment, this can influence how quickly the patient recovers. It is also important to blind patients, because their expectations can improve outcomes, and this can make a treatment appear effective when it isn't. If a patient knows they are getting the 'newest and best' drug they might expect to get better, and these expectations could cause an improvement (see Chapter Eight). Meanwhile, if the patient knows they are 'just' getting the placebo they might not have the same expectations. Placebo control treatments that patients think could be 'real' are used to help make sure blinding is applied and maintained during a trial. It also helps if other people involved in the trial, like the statisticians, are blinded since they too can introduce bias. But even if the blinding in an individual trial is perfect, it is not enough: we also have to avoid 'cherry picking'. Systematic reviews are a type of study used to help prevent cherry picking.

Systematic reviews to make a better final judgement

The Swiss Men's Ice Hockey team beat Canada in the 2006 Olympics. It would be wrong to say, on the basis of one game, that the Swiss team was better than the Canadian team. It is the only time they have ever beaten Canada in the Olympics, they have never won the Olympics, while Canada has won the Olympics nine times. To make a judgement about which is the best team, you need to look at the whole picture. Looking at the whole picture tells us that Canada has a much better team than Switzerland. The Swiss may have other advantages, like good chocolate, but in ice hockey they just aren't as good. The same applies to medical research, a fair assessment of whether a treatment 'wins' has to be based on all relevant evidence. As obvious as this seems, it happens more rarely than we might like.

If I wanted to know whether Prozac is more effective than a placebo, it would be wrong for me to cherry-pick my favourite studies that indicated a positive benefit of Prozac. It would be wrong to ignore those with a negative result. I'll give you an example of the harm caused when people ignore studies when I talk about 'publication bias' below. The first time I learned that we needed more than one study I was surprised – why isn't one enough? Either something works, or it doesn't, right? Wrong. That is only what headlines tell you. Anyone who has done real science knows that it is messy. There is a lot of randomness: once in a while a drug works with some people but not others, sometimes the study is flawed, and unfortunately researchers can cheat.

That is why it is so important to look at all the studies together in a mega study called a 'systematic review' to make sure you are not merely choosing the ones that give you the result you want. Once we have gathered all the trials together, it is sometimes possible to use statistical methods to get an average-effect size in what is called a 'meta-analysis'.

Summary: What is good evidence?

If there is a systematic review of blinded randomised trials showing that a treatment works, then it probably does. Otherwise we have reason to remain sceptical. Now you are probably asking whether there is good evidence showing that vitamin C can cure the cold, or whether marijuana cures depression. I just typed 'systematic review vitamin C cold' into Google, and learned that there is a systematic review of blinded randomised trials looking at the effects of vitamin C on colds. (I am not promoting Google as the ultimate scientific resource, I am telling you about it here to show that it can be quite easy to find a systematic review of randomised trials if you want to get a good idea about whether something works.)

I read the study carefully and its conclusions about vitamin C's effects are interesting. On the one hand, vitamin C does not seem to prevent colds. On the other hand, if you take vitamin C on a regular basis your cold will not last as long as it will if you do not take vitamin C. As for marijuana, a systematic review seems to suggest that it makes depression worse rather than better.

Some people will tell you there is a lot more to learn about evidence that medical interventions work than I have explained here, and they are right. You need an entirely different kind of evidence: qualitative research, to learn about people's feelings. You need to watch what happens to people for years to see what are the long-term effects of a treatment. Then, doctors will always need to use judgement to adapt evidence to individual patients, and we do not always need randomised trials or systematic reviews to prove treatments are effective. As I say, real science is messy, and it can also be depressing.

Three depressing things about medical studies

Publication bias
About half of trials are never published, especially those with negative results. This means that systematic reviews often contain a biased sample of trials, and often have exaggerated results. The unpublished trials are hard and sometimes impossible to find. In his TED Talk, Ben Goldacre talks about a time when he prescribed an antidepressant called reboxetine to one of his patients. Goldacre is an evidence guru so naturally he checked the literature and found that reboxetine had been proven superior to placebos and as good as other antidepressants. Because his patient had not responded to the other antidepressants, he decided to try reboxetine.

But it turns out that Ben did not have the full picture. There were six unpublished trials comparing reboxetine against placebo with negative results (where reboxetine was no better than placebo). There were also unpublished data comparing reboxetine with other antidepressants showing that reboxetine was *worse* than the other options. How can doctors and patients make good choices about treatments if trials are not published?

Worse, governments do not require that the drug companies release all data about benefits and harms. This is a kind of madness. What would you say if a company had suppressed information about the brakes in a car not working and people died in accidents as a result. I think the lack of any requirement for drug companies and others who do trials to release all the trial data on their products is crazy and most people I tell about this find it difficult to believe. The result is that doctors prescribe drugs without knowing how well they work or how serious the side effects are. If you are lucky enough to live in a country where they have socialised medicine, like Canada or the UK, then you pay for these treatments through your taxes. If you live in a country without socialised medicine, then you pay for them out of your pocket. You have the right to all the data about the benefits and harms of these treatments. Movements like the AllTrials campaign (www.alltrials.net) are fighting – with some success – to change this.

Hidden bias
It gets worse. Bias that cannot be detected can even fool people who are experts at judging whether tests are fair. The funny thing about these hidden biases is that they almost always support the new drug of the company that paid for the trial. Sometimes this leads to absurd conclusions. A research group in Germany looked at trials that compared three different antipsychotic drugs – olanzapine, risperidone and quetiapine – against each other. They found that olanzapine beat risperidone, risperidone beat quetiapine, and quetiapine beat olanzapine. But that is ridiculous.

What if I told you that Sarah was taller than Johnny, Johnny was taller than Mark, and Mark was taller than Sarah? It doesn't take too much brainpower to figure out that it cannot be true. Yet these kinds of Orwellian non-facts pervade the medical literature. The antipsychotic trials were all randomised and blinded, so they all looked as if they were trustworthy. The factor that appeared to determine the outcome was who paid for the study. When the manufacturers of risperidone paid for the trial, risperidone 'won', when the manufacturers of quetiapine paid, quetiapine 'won', and when the manufacturers of olanzapine paid, olanzapine won. Researchers in Germany conclude that the trials suffered from some 'hidden biases'. These 'hidden biases' are impossible to find by reading journal articles. Those articles can look squeaky clean, but questions must be asked about whether statistical tricks or outright cheating may have been used in the actual trial. Obviously this won't be reported in the journal article, so we don't know.

Size matters (and people lie about it)

Pound for pound, an ant is stronger than an elephant. A leafcutter ant can even carry something that weighs fifty times more than it. That is the equivalent of a human being lifting a truck with their teeth, or an elephant lifting a brick house. That is pretty incredible and I have a lot of respect for ants. But their pound-for-pound strength will not help me if I need to carry something heavy. For that, I would much prefer the help of an elephant (or a human). The geek name for pound-for-pound strength is relative strength, and relative things are even confused by smart humans with degrees from Harvard and Oxford. That is why, unless I say otherwise, I use absolute-effect sizes in this book. The good news is that if I tell you about the blue whale and the barnacle, I bet you will never get it mixed up again.

The blue whale is the largest known mammal ever to have lived on earth. Bigger than the biggest dinosaurs that we know of. Adult blue whales are about thirty metres long and weigh up to 170 tons. They are longer than two school buses parked end to end, their tails are as wide as a van, and their heart is as big as a small car. If you get very close to a blue whale, you will see tiny-shelled creatures called barnacles attached to its skin. Full-grown barnacles can easily fit into the palm of an adult's hand. Now if I asked you which creature had a bigger penis, the blue whale or the barnacle, you might think I was joking. The blue whale's is bigger than an adult human, while the barnacle's is barely longer than your hand. Clearly the blue whale wins. But that is only if we are talking absolute sizes.

If we are talking size relative to their body length, it is a different story. The barnacle's thingy is up to thirty times as long as its body. Barnacles do not move, so their penises have to be longer than their bodies to impregnate a mate. The blue whale's, on the other hand, is shorter than its body. So according to the relative measure, the barnacle's is larger than the blue whale's. When you read about medical treatment effects, they usually report relative not absolute-effect sizes, which can be confusing and misleading.

In the EUROPA study, investigators randomised 12,218 patients with heart disease to either take a drug called perindopril, or a placebo. Perindopril is a drug that relaxes blood vessels and lowers the amount of blood moving through the vessels so that the heart does not 'demand' as much blood. After taking the drug or placebo for over four years, investigators looked to see how many people who took perindopril died or had a serious heart attack, and compared that with what happened to the people who received the placebo. Ten per cent of the participants in the 'placebo' group died or had a serious heart problem, compared with eight per cent in the perindopril group. So the difference between the drug and the placebo was two per cent.

In some ways two per cent is a lot. It means out of one hundred people, you prevent two deaths or two heart attacks. To some people, two per cent is not very much. It means that you would have to give fifty people the drug to save one death or heart attack. When given the choice to take a pill every day for the rest of their lives, or have a two per cent reduced chance of heart attack or death, some will pop the pill. But many would choose to forget the pill and take their chances, or even try a little more exercise. (A systematic review of trials suggests that exercise may be as good as drugs for preventing heart disease.)

Then it gets confusing. The authors of the study did not say the drug had a two per cent effect, they said it had a twenty per cent effect. And because twenty per cent is very big, they said *everyone* at risk should take the drug. But how did they get twenty per cent from two per cent? They used the confusing relative-effect sizes. Saying perindopril reduced deaths and heart attacks by twenty per cent is like saying that a barnacle has a bigger penis than a blue whale. The mathematics required to calculate the relative-effect size is not too hard. You take the absolute size (two per cent) and divide it by the effect in the placebo group (ten per cent). In this case the relative-effect size is two per cent divided by ten per cent, which is twenty per cent.

With such a small absolute effect, a small hidden bias in the trial could have tipped it the other way. Here are two small things that might be relevant:

- All five members of the EUROPA executive committee declared a conflict of interest.
- More patients in the perindopril group dropped out, mostly because of negative side effects attributed to the drug. If these patients had not dropped out of the trial it might have made the apparent benefit of the drug even smaller.

One cannot help but wonder whether these things could have led to small hidden biases that influenced the results.

Because of this we should not be surprised if perindopril did not demonstrate superiority to placebo in another trial. In fact, that is just what happened.

37

In the PEACE study, investigators randomised 8,290 patients in four countries to receive trandolapril (a pharmaceutical cousin of perindopril) or placebo. Trandolapril failed to demonstrate superiority to placebo. The different results in the PEACE and EUROPA studies could be because the drugs were slightly different. It could also be because small effects in trials with hidden bias cannot be trusted.

A similar debate is going on now about statins. Statins are very effective for people who already have confirmed heart disease; for example, people who have already had a stroke or heart attack. But not everyone who takes statins has confirmed heart disease, and some experts say that everyone over forty (no matter what their risk of heart disease) should take them to prevent possible future disease. Yet statins are not very effective for people without confirmed heart disease.

In the most recent randomised trial of people without confirmed heart disease, 3.7 per cent of the people who took statins died over six years, while 4.8 per cent of the people who took the placebo died. This means that the (absolute) benefit of statins was 1.1 per cent (4.8 per cent minus 3.7 per cent). However, by the time the results got to press, they reported that statins reduced death by twenty-four per cent. How did they get twenty-four per cent from 1.1 per cent?

They used confusing relative effects . . .

Something else to consider is that the decision to take medicine is not just about benefits, but whether the benefits outweigh the harms. And it takes only a small harm to outweigh a small benefit. Small effects are also more likely to arise from small (hidden) biases. With that in mind, the following three facts are relevant:

- While statins are generally safe, some studies show about 1 in 100 people experience side effects like muscle pain or diabetes, and about 1 in 1,000 people will have a stroke.
- Other studies have concluded that there is a correlation

between financial conflicts of interest and effects of treatments being made bigger than they really are. Like the EUROPA example, many investigators who conducted the statin studies declared financial conflicts of interest, so questions have to be asked as to whether (consciously or unconsciously) they might have been affected by small (hidden) biases.

- The investigators who have completed the large statin trials have not released all the data, leaving questions about statins' overall benefits unanswered.

In spite of this, it is likely that statins do have some – albeit small – benefits for people who do not have confirmed heart disease. Faced with the choice to take a pill every day for the rest of their lives, or have a 1.1 per cent reduced chance of cardiovascular death, some will be happy to take the pill, while others might not.

Regardless of these problems with the statin evidence, some 'hard-core' statin believers say that we should not even be given the choice. Just like vitamins A and D used to be added to milk to prevent blindness and rickets, they say we should now pop statins like M&Ms. Or even add them to the water, so people are forced to take them. Especially in countries where there is a national health service and taxpayers pick up the tab to deal with heart attacks and strokes, why should we let people refuse to take statins if we are the ones who pick up the bill to treat them?

Small effects, they might add, are important if we add them up over the entire population. For instance, putting babies to sleep on their backs reduced infant deaths by much less than one per cent, but because so many babies are born, it probably saved over five hundred lives per year in the UK alone, and over two thousand lives per year in each of the US and Europe. Putting babies 'back to sleep' (as the campaigns were called) is a simple intervention that does save some babies' lives, and even one baby's life is important. Likewise, the reasoning goes, if everyone (even those with a low risk of heart disease) took statins, we would save thousands of lives.

The argument that we should be forced to take statins does not make much sense, because statins are not like vitamins A or D, or putting babies back to sleep. For one, there are other ways to reduce the risk of heart disease such as exercise and better diet, so forcing someone to take a statin takes away their freedom of choice. Also, the argument falls apart unless we are *sure* that (for people with a low or medium risk of heart disease) statin benefits actually outweigh the harms. The reality, as we have seen, is that there are a lot of open questions about whether the benefits outweigh the harms for people with a low or medium risk of heart disease. The problem with small effects is worse if we consider that average results don't always apply to individuals.

I am not average

My colleague and friend Professor Donald Gillies tells an interesting story about his niece in Rome. He was visiting his niece when she was about to turn sixteen. Apparently when teenagers in Rome turn sixteen, most of them get mopeds. Hoping to discourage his niece, Donald informed her about the evidence of the serious dangers of riding mopeds, such as paralysis and death. As an academic, Donald had studied the latest statistics, which he cited, hoping to scare his niece. To Donald's surprise, she immediately agreed with all the statistics. He thought he had succeeded at dissuading her from getting a moped. But then she added that the statistics did not apply to *her*. She said that the ones who were injured and died in moped accidents drove while drunk, drove too fast, and drove when they were too tired. She, on the other hand, rarely drank, would never drive too fast, and was generally very careful. She may not have known it, but she had stumped Donald with a major controversy in medicine: when do average results from trials apply to individuals?

Just as Donald's niece was different from the average Italian sixteen-year-old, you might be different from the average person in a clinical trial. Trials usually exclude smokers, people with more than one ailment, very young people, and very old people. Yet once a treatment is proven effective in a trial, it is used to treat everyone, even the people who would not have been eligible for the trial. But how do we know that the drug works in the people who were not eligible for the study? How do we know if the results of the trial apply to us? Well, sometimes they don't.

Some antidepressants proved to be effective when tested in adults, and were then used to treat children. However, later studies showed the drugs had doubtful effects in children. In a more dramatic case, an arthritis drug called benoxaprofen (Oraflex™ in the USA and Opren™ in Europe) proved effective in trials in 18–65-year-olds, but was withdrawn from the market immediately after it was reportedly responsible for deaths of 12 elderly patients who took the drug. There seemed to be something about older people's bodies that reacted with the drug in a fatal way.

The statin trials face a similar problem. The researchers conducting the trials excluded people with liver disease, muscle pain, patients taking other medications, and patients with any other 'serious condition(s) likely to interfere with study participation'. But many people who end up getting statins *are* taking other medications, have muscle pain, or liver problems. Just as Donald Gillies' niece said the evidence didn't apply to her, the results of the statin trials may not apply to many people who would have been excluded from the trial. The results certainly don't apply to all the people who would take them if statins were included in the water supply. For some individuals, the drug may be better than it was for the average person in the trial, and for others statins could be harmful.

Things get even more complicated if we think about national and cultural differences. A few years ago, an intervention designed to reduce malnutrition among children in Tamil

Nadu was introduced. The intervention involved educating mothers, additional healthcare, and food supplements. The intervention was a great success, with malnutrition declining by thirty-three per cent among children aged 6–24 months.

Inspired by the success in Tamil Nadu, a similar project was implemented in Bangladesh. However, the intervention did not work in Bangladesh. The people in Tamil Nadu and Bangladesh were not that different, but their culture was. Some of the reasons it didn't work in Bangladesh were what came to be called the 'mother-in-law' and 'man-shopper' factors. Unlike in Tamil Nadu, the mothers were not the decision-makers in Bangladesh. The men did the food shopping, so educating mothers did not have an effect on what was bought, and the mothers-in-law allegedly diverted the food supplements from the children to their sons.

There are different techniques for dealing with the problem that we might be different from the average person in a trial. All of them – most recently 'personalised medicine' and 'genetic medicine' – make huge promises, and consistently underdeliver. The details of the solutions can become somewhat esoteric, so I will not describe them here (see my papers on the problem of generalisability if you have an appetite for more geeky stuff). So, besides using the techniques for making sure that a treatment works for you, and not just the average person in a trial, it is important to monitor what happens to you when you take a new treatment. If it turns out that it is working, then great! It might even work better for you than it does for the average person in the trial.

On the other hand, if it doesn't work, or if you are getting side effects that (for you) do not outweigh the benefits, then you need to speak with your doctor about other possibilities. The problems with too much medicine suggest that this 'watch-and-see' attitude is not used enough.

Nothing (even a randomised trial) is perfect

When we hear about very large studies with thousands of people, we think this is a good thing and it usually is. Large trials are wonderful because differences between people 'wash out', making the trial more trustworthy. That is why randomised trials are considered to be the 'gold standard' of medical evidence. The irony is that we only need large studies when effect sizes are very small. You do not need to have a thousand races to figure out how fast Usain Bolt is compared to the competition, you need only a few.

Taking advantage of this irony, Gordon Smith and Jill Pell wrote a spoof article in 2003 called 'Parachute use to prevent death and major trauma related to gravitational challenge: a systematic review of randomised controlled trials' to poke fun at medical evidence experts. Smith and Pell concluded:

> Advocates of evidence-based medicine have criticised the adoption of interventions evaluated by using only observational [not from randomised trial] data. We think that everyone might benefit if the most radical protagonists of evidence-based medicine organised and participated in a double-blind, randomised, placebo-controlled, crossover trial of the parachute.

Smith and Pell are right that many treatments with huge effects do not need randomised trials. We know that automatic external defibrillation starts a stopped heart, tracheostomies open blocked air-passages, the Heimlich manoeuvre dislodges airway obstructions, penicillin cures pneumonia, and epinephrine cures severe anaphylactic shock. To the best of my knowledge none of these treatments have been tested in randomised trials, yet we know they work.

The problem is that all researchers and drug manufacturers think their new drug or treatment is so good that it does not need to wait for a big randomised trial before being used on

43

patients. However, in reality most of these treatments will not be revolutionary, and about half of new treatments turn out to be worse than the existing treatment. The only time we do not need randomised trials is when the *absolute*-effect size is really big, which is rare.

Conclusion

'Good' evidence is like a fair race – it is not that hard to understand if you avoid jargon. The problem is that most new treatment effects are tiny. So whenever you read about a breakthrough drug with a huge effect size, it is probably the relative effect. Like saying an ant is stronger than an elephant. In fact, a rule of thumb is that if you read a headline saying that a drug has a greater than ten per cent effect size, it is almost certainly the *relative*-effect size. There are many problems with evidence making it difficult to trust, so we have to remain sceptical. Just as democracy may be the worst system of government except for all the others, systematic reviews of blinded randomised trials are the best way we have to detect treatment effects, compared with all the others. The other methods often amount to little more than stories or opinion.

Takeaway 1: Ask your doctor about absolute benefits and harms

The next time you read something about a medical breakthrough or new diet or exercise regime, either from reading about it on social media or hearing it from your friends, do a little research. Is there a systematic review of randomised trials suggesting that it works? If there is no systematic review, is there one or more randomised trials? Is there evidence that it is harmful? Not everything you do has to be based on a systematic review of randomised trials, but you do need to ask some questions before believing things.

This is important because the chances are that at some point someone – either a medical professional or a media reporter – will try the relative-effect size trick on you. This is usually because they are confused themselves about the difference between absolute and relative risks. If anyone ever suggests that you take a treatment, you should ask:

- What will happen if you do not take the treatment?
- What benefit can you expect if you do take the treatment (what is the effect of the treatment – be sure to get the absolute-effect size)?
- What are the likely harms of the treatment?

Here is the kind of dialogue someone with a medium risk of cardiovascular disease might have with a doctor when discussing the possibility of taking statins. You can – and usually should – do the same exercise for any medication you or your children might take, especially painkillers, antidepressants, ADHC treatments and, as we will see in Chapter Seven, for knee, hip or back surgery.

To warn you in advance, I cannot tell you whether to take statins or some other treatment with a small average effect. The choice to take *any* treatment depends on the evidence and your values and circumstances, which are a matter of individual choice. This is a simple message yet it is often forgotten. For you to make the best choice about a treatment for *you*, you need to know about absolute-effect sizes and the harms. And to know whether the average effects apply to *you*, you need to monitor your progress. Here is an example of a dialogue someone considering statins might have with their doctor:

Doctor: According to your profile, you are considered to be at a medium risk of cardiovascular disease, which means you might have a heart attack or a stroke over the next ten years. Statins are recommended for people like you because they will reduce the chances of a fatal heart attack or stroke by about fourteen per cent.

You: Hmmm. If you don't mind, I have a few questions. First, what will happen if I don't take statins?

Doctor: Sure. Well, you are considered to be at a medium risk. In simple terms, this means that if we take one hundred people who are similar, about ten of you will have a serious heart attack or stroke in the next ten years if you don't take statins.

You: Thank you. Now I'd like to know what will happen if I do take statins. What are my chances of having a heart attack or stroke if I do take statins, in absolute terms?

Doctor: The latest evidence suggests that the absolute benefit of statins for people like you is between one per cent and two per cent. So whereas ten out of a hundred people like you are likely to have a stroke or heart attack in the next ten years if you *don't* take statins, only eight or nine of you would have a stroke or heart attack if you *do* take statins.

You: That makes sense. I have two more questions . . .

Doctor: Sure.

You: What are the likely harms of statins?

Doctor: Statins are quite safe for most people, and most people take them without experiencing side effects. That being said, about one in a hundred experience muscle pain or weakness; however, we aren't sure if the muscle pain and weakness is caused by the statins or that people simply feel pain and think it is because of the statins. They may also induce diabetes in about one in a hundred people. In very rare cases – about one in a thousand people – statin therapy may cause strokes.

You: Thanks. Now my last question. I've read some things on the internet about how evidence is biased. Is the evidence you are citing for statins biased?

Doctor: That is a good question, and it is true that a lot of evidence is biased. In the case of statins there has been controversy, because some of the scientists who have produced the statin data have declared financial conflicts of interest and have not released all the trial data. And in other cases where all the data has not been released and there are similar conflicts, we often end up learning that the benefits are exaggerated and the harms minimised. At the same time, a great deal of data has been published, so I don't think a closer independent look at the data will reveal any big surprises. We may find that the benefits are slightly lower than we thought and that the harms are ever so slightly greater; however, statins are still likely to have a benefit for people like you with a medium risk of cardiovascular disease.

At this point the patient can answer in one of three ways, so there are three possible endings to this dialogue . . . There is no absolute right or wrong here, there is only right or wrong for you, and you need answers to these questions to know what is best for you.

Ending 1: Not taking statins

You: Thank you, that makes sense. I think I'm going to hold off taking statins for now.

Doctor: That's fine. In that case I recommend that you keep up your exercise and stick to a healthy diet. And we can monitor you in our regular check-ups and see if your risk factors (and therefore the likely benefits of statins) change.

You: Thank you very much for your understanding. You have provided me with a good motivation to stick to my exercise regime and reduce the amount of dessert I eat.

Doctor: That's why I'm here, have a great day.

Ending 2: Taking statins

You: Thank you, I understand. Although the benefit is small, I'm happy to take a statin since it doesn't seem like a big deal to take the pills.

Doctor: That makes sense, many people don't see much of a downside and don't mind taking the pills. I still recommend that you keep up your exercise and stick to a healthy diet. We can re-evaluate at our next check-up.

You: Thank you very much for your understanding. I'll try to keep up with my exercise and good diet.

Doctor: You're welcome. Have a great day.

Ending 3: Wait and see

You: Thank you, that all makes sense. I think I need to think about it for a while.

Doctor: That's fine. I understand your scepticism about taking statins, and, to be clear, the choice is yours. Many people don't see much of a downside and don't mind taking the pills with their breakfast cereal, but others don't like taking pills. I'm going to give you the prescription anyway and you can choose whether or not to follow through with taking them. If you decide not to take them I recommend that you keep up your exercise and stick to a healthy diet. And we can monitor you. At some point if your risk level changes, we can re-evaluate what you'd like to do.

You: Thank you very much for your understanding. You have provided me with a good motivation to stick to my exercise regime and reduce the amount of dessert I eat.

Takeaway 2: Quick and easy way to check if there is a systematic review or randomised trial

To really confirm whether something works, you need to study critical appraisal and maybe even do another study. This can take years. But you can make a great guess that is likely to be correct by looking up whether there is a randomised trial or systematic review of randomised trials. Here are three ways, starting with the easiest, to look up whether there is a systematic review of randomised trials:

1. The easiest way is to Google it. For example, to find out whether marijuana cures depression, I typed in 'systematic review randomised trial marijuana depression'. I could not find anything. Then I typed in 'systematic review marijuana

depression' and found a systematic review, but it was not of randomised trials.

2. There are lots of websites that do the evidence search for you and summarise what they find in a user-friendly way. My favourite is one called 'NHS Choices', which is produced by the United Kingdom's National Health Service: http://www.nhs.uk/pages/home.aspx. I typed in 'depression', and did not find that they recommended marijuana for depression.

3. If you are feeling ambitious, you can go to the 'pubmed': https://www.ncbi.nlm.nih.gov/pubmed, which is a library of almost every medical trial or systematic review ever published. I typed in 'marijuana depression systematic review random*' and fourteen results popped up. (I put an asterisk after the word 'random' because you can spell randomised with an 's' or a 'z', and the asterisk tells PubMed to look for the word 'random' with any other ending.) One seemed relevant called 'Cannabinoids for Medical Use: A Systematic Review and Meta-analysis', and there was no high-quality evidence of a benefit of marijuana over placebo for depression.

Takeaway 3: Determine your cardiovascular risk, and what you can do to change it

This is a great website that will tell you what your risk of cardiovascular disease is and what you can do to change it: http://chd.bestsciencemedicine.com/calc2.html.

Have a look.

3
Beware of Stories and Expert Opinion

*An ounce of practice is generally worth more than a ton of
theory*

Ernst F. Schumacher

How empty is theory in the presence of fact!

Mark Twain

Ignaz Semmelweis was the Hungarian director of the maternity ward at the Vienna General Hospital in the 1840s. The
maternity ward was a big room divided into two halves called
Ward 1 and Ward 2. In Ward 1, doctors and medical students
– mostly male – delivered the babies. In Ward 2, midwives –
all female – delivered the babies. Semmelweis noticed that ten
per cent in Ward 1 were dying and fewer than four per cent
were dying in Ward 2.

He tried to figure out why so many mothers and babies
were dying in Ward 1. At the time, people believed the 'miasma
theory', an idea that diseases were caused by 'bad air'. This
was not as crazy as it sounds, because people were often ill
in crowded urban areas where the air was in fact very smelly.
In fact the word 'malaria' just means 'bad air' in Italian. But
Semmelweis realised the difference in maternal deaths could
not be bad air, because both wards were in the same room
with the same air.

The Viennese professors suggested it was foreign student
doctors who were causing the deaths because they were rough
with patients. Semmelweis agreed that the foreign doctors were
associated with more deaths, but it was because they worked
harder and treated more patients, not because they were less
well qualified or rough. Desperate, Semmelweis even persuaded

the priest, who normally walked through the first ward on the way to the second ward, to take a roundabout route and enter via the second ward. He thought the priest might frighten the patients into being more likely to die. The priest reluctantly agreed to change his point of entry, but deaths remained the same.

Then something very tragic happened to Semmelweis's colleague Jacob Kolletschka. While performing an autopsy, Kolletschka was accidentally stabbed in a finger by a student with a knife that had been used on the corpse. He soon became ill with the same symptoms as the mothers who were dying. Since Kolletschka's death and the mothers' deaths appeared to happen in a similar way, Semmelweis had a light-bulb moment. As it seemed that the doctor died because he was stabbed with a knife that had touched the dead body, maybe some particles from the dead body were reaching the mothers. But how? The autopsy room was in the basement, whereas the maternity wards were upstairs.

The link was simple: the doctors moved freely between the autopsy room and the maternity ward. They washed their hands with soap and water, but they did not disinfect their hands. Semmelweis thought that although the doctors washed their hands, some small particles from the dead bodies must be remaining under the doctors' fingernails. It seems obvious to us today that doctors should disinfect their hands after an autopsy before treating patients. But the reason it is evident *now* is because of what people like Semmelweis discovered!

To be sure, Semmelweis could not see the particles – he didn't have a powerful enough microscope; however, he instituted a policy of doctors and students washing hands with a solution of chlorinated lime, what we now call chlorine bleach, before entering the maternity ward.

Soon after the students started disinfecting their hands, the death rates in Ward 1 reduced to below the death rates in Ward 2. Very happy, Semmelweis wrote about his discovery in a book, and in medical publications across the world. His work eventually became very famous, with his name on coins, stamps, and even a university named after him in his native Budapest.

But all his fame came after he died. At the time, the reaction to Semmelweis was hostile. The other famous doctors in Europe rejected Semmelweis's findings. A British doctor called James Young Simpson said that the Brits already knew about Semmelweis's discovery. This was untrue, because sixty per cent of people who had surgery in London hospitals died of postoperative infections. Semmelweis's Viennese colleagues also rejected his policy of disinfecting hands. He was demoted and forbidden from treating patients. More women in Ward 1 quickly started dying again.

Disgusted, Semmelweis went back to Budapest, where he began drinking and slowly going insane. He was forced into an asylum where he was severely beaten by guards, secured in a straightjacket and confined to a dark cell. He died two weeks later from a gangrenous wound, possibly caused by the beating.

How could Semmelweis's live-saving discovery have been rejected? Some believe it was because he was a Hungarian in Vienna, and the Austrians might have been prejudiced against him. This prejudice may have mattered in Vienna itself, but not elsewhere in Europe where his work was published. The latest research suggests the reason for his failure was that he did not have a theory to explain how disinfecting hands could work. His colleagues didn't know about germs and did not understand how a tiny amount of material from the corpses could cause the mothers to die. Their refusal to believe Semmelweis's observations was due to their obsession with a theory (which Semmelweis didn't have).

A few years after Semmelweis died, Joseph Lister did some experiments proving that germs caused disease supported by the 'germ theory' of disease, disinfecting hands became (and still is) one of the most important things that all doctors learn to do. Did you know that the mouthwash 'Listerine' comes from Lister?

Too much focus on theory over observations can be dangerous for introducing new treatments, too. Indeed, before modern medicine, most treatments such as bloodletting and leeching fell into this category. Bloodletting was based on the theory of the four humours. According to this theory, our bodies contained four humours: blood, phlegm, yellow bile, and black bile. Diseases (again according to this theory) were caused when these four humours were out of balance.

Blood was thought to be the dominant humour, so when people were ill, it was often believed to be because there was too much blood. The cure, therefore, was to cut the person to release some blood (usually about half a litre). The most prominent medical journal in the UK is *The Lancet*. 'Lancet' is the name of the knife used to cut the person to let blood. Ironically, bloodletting probably had a huge placebo effect, so it might have made people feel better, at least temporarily. At the same time it was almost certainly harmful for many of the diseases it was intended to treat. George Washington was probably bled to death by his four doctors.

Here is a more recent example of a bad theory leading to a harmful treatment. Irregular heartbeats called arrhythmias are known to increase the chances that someone dies from a heart attack. So when drugs that reduced irregular heartbeats were discovered, they gave them to people having attacks. The theory was that reducing irregular heartbeats would also reduce death after heart attacks. On this basis, hundreds of thousands of people were given the drugs. However, some American cardiologists insisted on doing a trial comparing the drugs against placebos. Proponents of the drugs thought those taking the placebo would die. The trial began in 1987, and 1,727 patients were randomised to receive the drugs or placebo.

The results? Researchers analysed the outcomes halfway through the trial and found that eight out of ten people taking the drug died, but only three out of ten people in the placebo group died. They concluded that it was the drugs not the placebos that were killing people. Based on these results, they stopped the trial early and the drugs were withdrawn as a treatment for irregular heartbeats. More than 50,000 people who took the drugs died each year, which is more than the total number of Americans who died in the Vietnam War.

Theories are important for helping us find new things to test in randomised trials, and stories are useful for teaching and remembering. And some theories or stories about treatments will turn out to be supported by evidence, but many will not and we cannot be sure until we actually test them. A problem is that experts often support theories or stories without checking the evidence. We have to remember that just because someone is an expert, it does not make them right.

Being an expert does not make you right

I remember the first time I went to a medical conference as an invited speaker. I had just finished my PhD in philosophy. At philosophy conferences, they used to put us up in student dorms and give us sandwiches for lunch. So I was surprised when I was put up in a fantastic five-star hotel and given lavish meals at the medical conference. (It was an academic conference, not an industry conference, by the way.)

I was so surprised that I told a senior medical colleague how great it was compared to philosophy conferences. His response was (I am withholding his name so I don't slander him, he was a nice guy): 'Jeremy, this is nothing. You should have seen in the 1990s before strict rules about taking money from pharma came into effect. They used to fly me and my family first class to the south of France, we'd have a meeting in the morning, go to the beach in the afternoon, and all we'd have to do is sign up to a consensus statement at the end.'

The consensus statement was then used as 'proof' that the new treatment worked. Until the emergence of the EBM movement, 'consensus statements' were the main way of deciding whether treatments worked. That is why Trish Greenhalgh called the consensus method the GOBSAT method, which stands for 'Good Old Boys Sat Around a Table'. The conflict of interest and industry bias has not disappeared. However, at least now the experts must produce or refer to evidence to support their views.

Sir Iain Chalmers, who founded the Cochrane Collaboration, (a group that specialises in producing systematic reviews) tells another interesting story about why we cannot trust what 'experts' say, or trust stories about how things work. He was working at a refugee camp in the Gaza Strip, and saw many children with measles. Now measles is a viral disease, so antibiotics do not work. And he had been told again and again by his expert teachers at medical school not to give antibiotics to treat viral infections such as measles. So he conserved his limited supply of antibiotics and did not give it to children with measles. The children were often malnourished or in poor health and had other complications. Sadly, some of them died a few days after Iain saw them.

Iain's Palestinian colleague was seeing very similar children with measles, but almost none of the children he treated died. After a year or so, one of the Palestinian doctors gently pointed out to Iain that giving antibiotics to the children with measles helped, because these vulnerable children often developed bacterial infections in addition to measles. Iain changed his practice and started prescribing antibiotics to children with measles, and noticed that the children were less likely to die. This experience taught Iain to be very sceptical of what he was told by 'experts', and he began a lifelong crusade to insist on good evidence.

Iain's experience is not isolated. Textbook recommendations (written by experts) for treatments intended for heart attack often do not mention the latest advances. In some cases they keep recommending treatments long after they have proven to be harmful, or fail to recommend treatments that have proved to be effective! If we add that many experts have a conflict of interest because they are paid by industry, there is even less reason to trust experts.

Unfortunately, the problem with researchers who produce the evidence having financial conflicts of interest is a very common one. A recent study of the most influential experts within the American Psychiatric Association (APA) showed that many of its members had declared being paid by the pharmaceutical industry. Given that many of these experts are often involved in deciding what is an 'official' psychiatric disorder, and what is not, this raises questions about some of the more controversial classifications which have been made.

Until 1973 the APA classified homosexuality as a disease, and in their most recent report they branded a bunch of things that most of us would consider normal differences between people to their list of 'diseases'. Besides the adult attention deficit disorder already mentioned above, they have named Restless Leg Syndrome (a desire to move one's legs) and Caffeine Intoxication Disorder (a 'disease' you have if you get excited after having three or four cups of coffee). Most people I know get excited after drinking three straight cups of coffee and many people I know sometimes move their legs.

Now the odd person may have such a severe case that they need serious treatment, but the vast majority are just human. How did these normal things get classified as diseases? Did the conflicts of interest play a part in the classification of these apparently normal things as diseases? It is a fair question, given that most of the experts who have promoted these normal things as diseases have declared ties to the same companies that make the medications used to treat the disorders.

Psychiatry is not the only industry with rampant conflicts of interest. As I described in the section on hidden bias, these financial conflicts of interest have been shown time and time again to influence results, often in ways that are difficult to detect.

But in the end, what can we trust?

Okay, I can hear you think, in the last chapter you said systematic reviews of randomised trials are great, but hidden biases and other stuff make them hard to trust. Now you are saying that people in studies are different from us and that we cannot trust theories or experts either. So what *can* we trust?

The answer to this question is that we have to keep asking questions, but it is not all doom and gloom either. We *are* different from the average person in a trial because we are unique, yet human bodies are also similar in a lot of ways and many treatments work for most people. And even though stories and experts are problematic, they can still be useful in many cases – especially when supported by evidence. And while there are problems with systematic reviews of randomised trials, they are better than the alternatives.

If we remain sceptical and do a bit of work to find good evidence, then we can often be quite confident that a treatment is better than a placebo. This brings us to the question: how powerful are placebos?

Takeaway: Check if there is evidence for what the expert or story says

About once per week someone I know tells me about a new diet or exercise routine or food supplement they swear has changed their lives. They are often based on bestselling books, or beautiful experts who are producing lots of YouTube videos. If I am totally honest, I have tried some stuff myself. Most of these things are unlikely to hurt you, and a lot of them work because of the placebo effect. It is still important to check the evidence for two reasons:

- The treatments might be harmful.
- You might be able to do something even better.

So let's go over a conversation between me and someone who recently told me about a diet where they were supposed to drink just pomegranate juice (and eat nothing else) for ten days. It is a true story. I will call the person who told me about this diet Sabrina:

> **Sabrina:** Have you heard of this new fasting diet called the pomegranate diet? You just eat pomegranate and nothing else for three days. It is supposed to clean your system, boost your immune system, and make your skin shine.
>
> **Jeremy:** I haven't heard of it, but it sounds interesting. Do the people promoting it provide you with any evidence?
>
> **Sabrina:** Yes, it has been tested on people at a research university. And they explain how it works [the story]. Basically, pomegranate is a superfood. It has a lot of vitamin C, which can boost your immune system. And fasting cleans out stuff that gets stuck in your system. This all makes your body cleaner and healthier.
>
> **Jeremy:** Well, there are three things you are asking about. First, is fasting good for health? Second, are pomegranates good for health? And third, is fasting on pomegranate good for health?
>
> **Sabrina:** I suppose, yes.
>
> **Jeremy:** Well, most cultures and religions have some kind of fasting and have been doing it for thousands of years. So I doubt very much that fasting in general is deadly (unless you do something really dumb like stop drinking anything for days, or stop eating altogether for months). But let's check the evidence.
>
> **Sabrina:** Okay.

Jeremy types 'systematic review randomised trial fasting' into Google for a 'quick and dirty' search. He finds a systematic review supporting the benefits of fasting.

Jeremy: Obviously a complete investigation would take years. However, a quick search shows there are a few systematic reviews of what is called 'intermittent fasting', which means on-and-off fasting. It seems that there is likely to be a health benefit, but more evidence is required.

Sabrina: Good!

Jeremy: Well, hold on, just because fasting in general is good, it doesn't mean that pomegranate fasting is good.

Sabrina: True.

Jeremy: The next thing I'm going to check is whether pome-granates are good for our health . . . *Pauses to search* . . . Again, this is a quick search so we can't be one hundred per-cent sure. However, one systematic review shows that pomegranates can help lower blood pressure, and weaker evidence shows that it can slow the progress of prostate cancer. I didn't find any evidence that pomegranates cause any damage.

Sabrina: See, I told you!

Jeremy: Well, hold on again, just because fasting is good and pomegranates are good, it doesn't mean that fasting on pomegranates is good.

Sabrina: Okay. You academic types can be really annoying sometimes.

Jeremy: *Pauses to search* . . . I couldn't find any randomised trials or systematic reviews of pomegranate fasting.

Sabrina: Hmm.

Jeremy: That doesn't mean it is bad, it just means there is no evidence.

Sabrina: So what is the bottom line?

Jeremy: Well, based on what we know, it probably won't harm you. And eating pomegranates as part of a regular diet seems good for you. However, to fast on pomegranates alone means you would be experimenting on yourself like a guinea pig.

Sabrina: What should I do?

Jeremy: Well, I can't tell you what to do, I can just share two things that might help you make a decision. First, you can go with the intermittent fasting method that is recommended by the systematic review. Or, if you want to try something not supported by a randomised trial, at least choose something that has stood the test of time rather than something promoted by a small group of people who haven't used it for long enough even to use their experience to measure the long-term effects. I can tell you what I will do.

I fast from time to time, for example at the beginning of Lent, and as part of my yoga discipline. However, when I do this I am using methods that have existed for thousands of years, which means that while there are no randomised trials, there is a wealth of casual observational data and experience. I also surround myself with experts who have done the type of fasting I'm doing. So if I feel funny, or something goes wrong, I can ask an expert.

Many Christians fast before Easter and a priest might tell you what the best recipes are and guide you. Muslims fast during Ramadan and they have experts, and there are traditional Indian yogis who have been doing various types of fasting who could also guide you. Why choose something new that might be great, but could also be harmful, and might not be as good as what's been around for centuries where you can get proper guidance?

Sabrina: That makes sense. I might try a more traditional method of fasting, and add pomegranates into my regular diet. Thanks for your advice!

Jeremy: You are welcome! And thank you for asking the question because I've learned something, too. I've learned that pomegranates probably have a health benefit, at least for lowering blood pressure. I happen to like how they taste, too, so I'm going to eat more of them.

4
Powerful Placebo Effects

*Three factors are of major importance in the suffering of
badly wounded men [during the Second World War]: pain;
mental distress; and thirst. Therapy has been almost entirely
directed to pain, and this usually limited to the administration of morphine in large dosage.*

Henry Knowles Beecher,
American anaesthetist and medical ethicist

The American anaesthetist Henry Knowles Beecher put his
academic career on hold to serve in the US Army during the
Second World War. While working on the frontline in southern
Italy, he reportedly saw something extraordinary. With supplies
of pain-killing morphine running out, a nurse injected a
wounded soldier with saltwater instead of morphine before
an operation. The soldier thought it was real morphine, and
it seemed to work: the soldier did not appear to feel any pain.
Beecher is said to have continued the practice, and returned
to the US convinced of the power of placebos.

While there are no historical records to confirm this
often-repeated account, in 1955 Beecher carried out a systematic review of fifteen previous studies (with over 1,000
patients) that had groups of patients who received placebos
in them. He found that a third of patients who receive
placebos got better. He published his findings in a widely
cited paper called 'The Powerful Placebo'.

One confusing thing about Beecher's study is that we do
not know if it was the placebos (like saltwater) that made
the patients get better or it was the body's self-healing ability
at work independently of the placebo treatments. After all,
many common illnesses like colds and flu clear up no matter

what we do. The medical term for something going away on its own is 'natural history'. (Geeky aside: philosophers call the mistaken inference that placebos have cured a condition based on some people getting better after receiving placebo the *post hoc ergo procter hoc* fallacy: after, therefore because of, fallacy.)

Many people have written about Beecher, debating how powerful placebos really are. Some say placebos are even more effective, and one major study coming out of Denmark claims that placebos have hardly any effect at all. I led a team of researchers to do a systematic review that helped to resolve this controversy. To do this, we compared the size of placebo effects with the size of 'real' treatment effects. Our review contained 152 trials (containing over 15,000 patients), and we found that *on average* placebos have almost the same effect sizes as 'real' treatments.

The overall effect of a treatment is a combination of both the placebo effect *and* the drug effect, so we would not always want to replace treatments with placebos. Say that someone ranks their pain at 5 on a scale of 0–10 (where 0 is no pain and 10 is worst pain imaginable). If we gave that person a placebo treatment, their pain might be reduced from 5 to 4. If we then gave that person a drug, their pain would be reduced from 4 to 3. So taking the drug would have a bigger effect than taking the placebo alone, even though the drug effect compared to placebo is the same as the placebo effect compared to nothing. You can still often – but not always (see the antidepressant example below) – get an additional benefit from the treatment. That being said, you can also get additional *harms* from the drugs: placebos are generally much safer than 'real' treatments. What is more, if we construe placebo effects more broadly to include expectations, empathy and other things I talk about in this book, we get an even larger placebo effect. This means that there are many common ailments for which placebo treatments are the best and safest option.

As I did my research, I learned that there are many misconceptions about placebos and placebo effects. The biggest one is that placebos are 'inert' substances – basically annoying noise that needs to be controlled in a trial, or something that quacks use to sell their snake oil. Placebos are neither inert, nor inactive, nor nonspecific. They are active, and their effects can be as specific as 'real' treatments. When the patient expects to get better after taking a placebo painkiller, their body will produce its own morphine (endorphins), which is as active and specific as the morphine that a doctor might inject.

I also learned and have written in my academic work about two other cool things about placebos that I had not thought about previously:

- Placebos come in many different forms. There are placebo pills, tablets, injections, and even sham surgery (more about that in Chapter Ten). They also come in different colours.
- Different placebos have different effects. In general, the more invasive the placebo, the more effective it is. So, two pills have greater effects than one pill, placebo injections have bigger effects than placebo pills, placebo acupuncture has a bigger effect than placebo injections, and sham surgery has the biggest effect of all. Different colour placebos also have different effects, with red placebos having more of a stimulant effect than blue ones, which have a depressive effect.

In fact, sometimes all that is required for a placebo effect is for a doctor to watch someone, in which case it is called a Hawthorne effect.

Hawthorne effect: when doing nothing is something

In a series of experiments between 1924 and 1933, scientists fiddled with the lighting in parts of the Hawthorne works belonging to the Western Electric Company factory near Chicago. When they turned the lights up in one part of the factory, they found that productivity went up. Then they tried turning the lights down: productivity went up again. They kept playing with different light intensities until the lights went so low that workers said they couldn't see and production unsurprisingly dropped. Since productivity increased whether the lights were turned up, turned down, or remained the same, they reasoned this outcome was not related to the change in lighting. Eventually the researchers worked out that productivity was increasing because the workers knew they were part of an experiment and worked harder. Scientists called the effect of being observed the Hawthorne effect. Something similar can happen to patients in clinical trials.

When a patient is in a trial, they are usually observed carefully by doctors. Knowing that they are being monitored, the patients might do things that are good for their health like exercise more, eat healthier, drink less alcohol, or simply expect to recover. These could all produce positive effects. The contact that patients have with healthcare practitioners could also have a positive effect (more on this in Chapter Ten). Confirming the likelihood of Hawthorne effects within medical trials, a systematic review found that even patients who are untreated (for example, they are on the waiting list for a trial) improved by twenty-four per cent.

More reasons to believe in placebo effects

Selective serotonin reuptake inhibitors (SSRIs) and the doctor effect

SSRIs are a class of antidepressant drugs that includes Prozac, Zoloft, and Luvox. With around one in ten adults in developed nations taking them to help reduce symptoms of depression, these drugs have made drug companies billions of dollars. According to the 'serotonin theory', depression is caused by the lack of a brain-signalling chemical called serotonin. SSRI drugs do not actually produce serotonin, but they prevent the body from absorbing it once it has been produced, so that more serotonin ends up in the body, thereby reducing the symptoms of depression. And many people who take SSRIs report feeling much better. But here is the rub: placebos work almost as well as SSRIs for people with mild or moderate depression.

People with mild or moderate depression have some, but not all, of the symptoms of depression:

- Persistent low mood and feelings of sadness, with or without weepiness
- Marked lack of interest in previously pleasurable activities
- Sleep pattern disturbances
- Change in appetite
- Tiredness
- Sluggish movements or agitation
- Difficulty in concentrating or solving simple everyday problems
- Feelings of guilt and/or worthlessness

The symptoms must persist for at least two weeks, in such a way that they affect the ability to function normally and they cannot be due to some other reason. People with severe depression have all or almost all the symptoms. When Irving Kirsch did a review of forty-seven previous trials comparing SSRIs with placebos, he found that unless a person was severely depressed, the difference between the drugs and the placebos was so small it would be hard for a depressed person to detect. Kirsch's study (and others like it) have even led some scientists to believe that the 'serotonin theory' is mistaken, and that depression isn't really linked to serotonin.

The main point here is not about serotonin, it is that the trials seem to show that placebos seem to be quite good for treating depression. Does this mean that we could or should give mildly depressed people Tic Tacs instead of drugs?

Probably not, because we do not believe in the power of Tic Tacs as much as we believe in drugs, so Tic Tacs would be unlikely to have the same benefits. However, for many people with mild to moderate depression, a doctor (or patient) familiar with all the aspects of self-healing and placebo effects that I present in this book is likely to have the same antidepressant benefits as a drug, and without the side effects or risk of dependence.

Active placebos are more effective than standard placebos (note to reader: this section gets a bit nerdy, so feel free to skip it)
Even when researchers try to keep a trial blind, patients in trials are quite good at detecting whether they have got the real thing or the placebo. This is because it can be really hard to make placebo treatments that look, taste and smell exactly like the real drugs. And some studies show that even if researchers try their hardest to keep a trial blinded, more than half of the participants can guess whether they are taking the placebo or not. Even if patients cannot tell the difference at the beginning of the trial, they sometimes get side effects and so realise immediately that they are taking the 'real' treatment.

For instance, a common side effect of tricyclic antidepressants is dry mouth. Patients in tricyclic antidepressant trials who get a dry mouth might realise they are receiving the 'real' intervention and develop a positive expectation about recovery. Meanwhile those who do not experience dry mouth may realise they are receiving only a placebo, causing them to have negative expectations. I will explain in Chapter Eight how negative expectations about a treatment can cause worse outcomes.

To get around this problem, researchers sometimes put chemicals into placebos so that they cause the same side effects as drugs. These 'active placebos' are better at tricking patients into believing that they are getting the real thing. Psychiatrist Joanna

Moncrieff and colleagues at University College London compared the effects of active and standard placebos in trials in which they were up against antidepressants. Active placebos had greater effects than normal placebos.

Summary: How powerful are placebos?

Placebos are not a panacea for everything, yet like 'real' medicine, placebos work quite well for some things. Also, placebos are not just pills. They can be injections, sham surgery (more about this in Chapter Ten), or funny-tasting drinks (more about this in Chapter Nine). We will also see in the upcoming chapters that you do not need placebo treatments to have placebo effects. Moreover, placebos are less likely to harm patients, and doctors who exploit placebo effects (either on their own or in addition to effective treatments) will have better outcomes than doctors who do not. But if placebos work, why can't you get a prescription for one? Typical answers to this question no longer make sense.

Why it is ethical to use placebos

The main reason doctors hesitate to give placebos is that they believe it requires them to lie to their patients. Recent studies suggest this is not true. Ted Kaptchuk, Professor of Medicine at Harvard Medical School, conducted a placebo-controlled trial for people with severe irritable bowel syndrome (IBS). Those for whom normal treatment was not working were randomised either to a waiting list, or to be given pills they knew were placebos. (I will solve the mystery of how these 'open-label placebos' work in Chapter Nine.) The placebos were presented to patients as: 'placebo pills made of an inert substance, like sugar pills, that have been shown in clinical studies to produce significant improvement in IBS symptoms through mind-body self-healing processes'. Kaptchuk found this type of placebo to have a similar effect as many 'real' drugs for IBS (although the existing therapies were not all that effective either).

Linda Buannono was a woman who took part in the trial, had been suffering from IBS for years and nothing had helped. Some days she was in so much pain she could barely leave the house. The open-label placebo had a great positive benefit. So much so that she said, 'I never felt better in my life.' But then at the end of the trial she stopped receiving the placebos and her IBS became worse again. A pharmacist whom she asked for some placebos said he was unable to give her any because it would be unethical.

Kaptchuk's trial using placebos that people *knew* to be placebos shows that there is no need for doctors to deceive their patients. We also do not need to give someone a placebo to have placebo effects. As we saw with the Hawthorne effect, simply paying attention to someone can improve their symptoms, and as we will see in the upcoming chapters, positive messages and empathetic care can also induce placebo effects without any inherent deception.

So, placebos are sometimes a good option and we need not lie, and in those cases there are no good ethical objections. It is hardly surprising then that surveys carried out in many different countries show most doctors have used placebos. Instead of worrying about how to ban them, we need to explore ways to expand their use in an ethical way.

A final problem people have with placebos is that they say placebos might work for others, but not for them. They say things like, 'placebos might work for naïve, gullible, uneducated people, but I am rational and smart and nobody fools me, so placebos won't work for me'. While it is true that placebos (like 'real' treatments) work for some people but not others, we cannot predict who they will work for. So even people who *think* placebos won't work for them could be surprised.

In fact, our beliefs about ourselves are often mistaken. If you ask people whether they are better-than-average drivers, most say yes. But as long as we make a nerdy statistical assumption that the distribution is not skewed (which we can), only half of us can be better than average. The other half are worse than average.

Likewise, if you ask people if they can tell the difference between expensive and cheap wine, most say yes, whereas hundreds of studies show that only a small handful of people actually can. With placebos it is similar: it is hard to tell who placebos will work for. Some studies are starting to show that placebos appear to be most effective for those who are more suggestible, those who are more optimistic, and those in whom brain structures associated with pleasure are more sensitive to placebo effects. But the studies are not definitive, so for now we cannot predict exactly who will respond to placebos.

All this is to say that since placebos work, we do not need to lie to patients to use them, and doctors should exploit placebo effects more. We can also exploit placebo effects for ourselves (see the takeaway exercise at the end of this chapter). This brings us to the question of how placebos work.

How do placebos work?

There are many different types of placebos that can work in different ways, and you do not need placebo treatments to have placebo effects. So we cannot really say how placebos work without talking about what kind of placebos we are talking about. However, in general, most placebos work in three main ways:

- Doctor healing effects. When a doctor makes us feel less anxious, this can lower our pain and reduce depression (see Chapter Ten).
- Expectations. When we expect something good to happen (like getting better), the brain's reward system is activated, triggering the production of the body's own painkilling

drugs like endorphins. This is what some call the 'power of belief' (see Chapter Eight where I describe my systematic review of expectation effects).

- Conditioning. Even if we do not consciously expect something to happen, our immune systems may be conditioned to react in certain ways when a doctor gives us a placebo pill (see Chapter Nine).

Also, being treated by an empathetic doctor can reduce stress and help us relax, which can have additional health benefits (see Chapters Eight and Nine).

Takeaway (for everyone): The 'Best Possible Self' exercise to boost the power of expectations

I have adapted this technique from the 'positive psychology' movement. Systematic reviews suggest it is quite good for anxiety-related disorders and depression. The cool thing about positive psychology is that if you have a 'mental illness', they do not focus on it. Instead, they try to focus your attention on personal growth and what it means to have a meaningful, happy life. You will need about thirty minutes to complete this exercise, and you will need a pen and some paper:

1. Think about a time in the future, for example six months, one year, five years.
2. For ten minutes write continuously about what your best life in that future time would look like. Visualise yourself in the best possible way – your dream life. Don't worry about grammar and do not stop moving the pen, and imagine the brightest possible future for yourself. Try to be as specific as possible. Express yourself without holding back, and at the same time avoid fantasies to focus on things that are achievable in the 'best-case' or 'good-case' scenario.
3. Once you have written for ten minutes, take a pause. Think whether there are any additional details you would

like to add. If so, add them. Again, be as specific as possible.

4. Now look at what you have written and reflect. Think of the 'future you'. What character strengths does this future version of you possess?
5. What character strengths do you think you need to make the future you described a reality? Write these down. Ask yourself, 'What would I be doing right *now* if I had that character strength?' Do it.

Here is a very short version of a 'best possible life' story: 'I envision spending quality time with my family and having amazing vacations together. The character trait I see in that picture is "prudence", and that's just what I'll need to enhance my financial situation in a way that maintains my work/life balance so that I can spend time with my family. If I had that kind of prudence *now* I would pay off and cancel all my credit cards so that I never pay high interest rates.'

Takeaway (for doctors): Exploit the placebo effect

Some studies suggest that 'alternative' practitioners are much better at doing so than conventional doctors, but all doctors can (and should) exploit placebo effects. No matter how serious the illness, you can enhance the effectiveness of your interaction by being positive and empathetic. I will describe the details of how this is done in Chapters Eight, Nine and Ten. If you have a patient with a complaint that you are sure does not require any 'real' medicine, and they refuse to go away until you give them something, then in addition to being positive (Chapter Eight) and empathetic (Chapter Ten), you can offer them something harmless such as vitamin C (or some other vitamin, after verifying that it will not harm the patient, perhaps by inducing an allergic reaction).

You do not need to lie to the patient. You can say something like Kaptchuk told his IBS patients: 'These vitamin C tablets are pills that don't have a specific effect for your problem; however, pills like these have been shown in clinical studies to produce significant improvement in [*you fill in the blank*] symptoms through mind-body, self-healing processes.'

PART II
Fight, Flight, Feed and Breed

It's very important that we relearn the art of resting and relaxing. Not only does it help prevent the onset of many illnesses that develop through chronic tension and worrying; it allows us to clear our minds, focus, and find creative solutions to problems.

Thich Nhat Hanh,
Vietnamese Buddhist monk and peace activist

Our bodies are extraordinary self-healers. Humans are also good at defending themselves against germs and viruses, and fighting wolves. Both self-healing and self-defence help us survive. The problem is that they also work against each other. When you have to fight a wolf, it is helpful to divert all your blood supply to things you need to fight, such as your arms and legs. But that additional blood supply has to get diverted from somewhere else. It comes from things that you do not need during a fight like the digestive system and the immune system. The way you burn energy also changes. In the fight-or-flight state, your body puts extra sugar into your blood for a quick energy-fix. But this comes from an adjustment in pancreatic fluid that leads to less fat being burned, and more fat on your belly and increased risk of heart disease. Basically, the things that are great for fighting a wolf are not always good for your health.

We have all experienced the fight-or-flight response so can empathise with it. Imagine you are celebrating a special occasion with a loved one at a really nice restaurant. The lighting is low and you are feeling romantic, and you also feel a bit hungry. Suddenly a psycho storms into the room with a gun. Your hunger and romantic desire vanish in an instant, because all your inner resources prepare you to run or fight, and eating and romance can get in the way of that. Later, after the intruder is removed and you are able to relax, you might feel hungry and sexy again. That is why the opposite of the 'fight-or-flight' response is called the 'feed-and-breed' response.

Stress, which is like a mini fight-or-flight response, is not always a bad thing. The problem is that most of us have too much stress, so our body's fight-or-flight response gets activated too often. It probably will not surprise you that stress is a risk factor for diseases ranging from depression to heart disease. Unfortunately, modern life is stressful, so high levels of stress are hard to escape. The good news is that we can manage our stress levels in two ways. First, by adopting different ways of thinking, we can change how our bodies react to the things that stress us out. Second, we can lower our stress levels by finding ways to relax and activate our feed-and-breed responses.

5
The Stress Response

I have been through some terrible things in my life, some of which actually happened.

Mark Twain

I've missed more than 9,000 shots in my career. I've lost almost 300 games. 26 times, I've been trusted to take the game winning shot and missed. I've failed over and over and over again in my life. And that is why I succeed.

Michael Jordan

How your body reacts to a wolf attack

Imagine you are a caveman. It is the dawn of human history and you have been out all day hunting. On the way home, you and your friends accidentally startle a pack of wolves. They growl as you pick up a stone to throw at them. You have not moved far, but inside your body a lot is happening. Anticipating a brawl, your body's 'fight-or-flight' alarm system goes off. Adrenaline and cortisol are pumped into your veins to boost energy levels. Your blood pressure and heart rate jump to send more oxygen to your muscles. Your pupils dilate so you can see better in the dark. The vessels in your lungs dilate so you can take in more oxygen. Pancreatic levels are adjusted to give you more quick-fix sugar energy in your blood. The pain-message system in the brain gets suppressed so that pain will not stop you defending yourself.

This astonishing response is great for helping you survive dangerous encounters. In your state of heightened alertness, you hurl a stone at the wolves. This time you are lucky. They growl then retreat. You let out a sigh as your whole body relaxes. You walk back to camp, where you enjoy an evening by the fire. Life as a Neanderthal is physically hard, but predictable. Accidental encounters with wolves are rare.

Jump forward to today. To this morning. You awake startled as the alarm on your smartphone drags you away from a pleasant dream. While prodding the screen to make the incessant beeping stop, you notice a calendar reminder about the meeting you have later with your boss. That means either good or bad news about your bonus – which you need to take the holiday by the sea that you have been looking forward to. Despite leaving early, a traffic jam delays your journey.

Your boss is angry when you turn up late and warns you that you can forget about your bonus if you are late again. He hands you a stack of files and tells you to go through them before lunch. You grip your coffee mug a little tighter as you momentarily indulge the fantasy of hurling it at your boss. In reality, you swallow, look down, and get back to work. Back at your desk, you feel a stabbing pain in your back caused by an old sporting injury. Regular exercise usually helps, but there is no time for that now, so you reach into your drawer for a few painkillers. You feel tired so you make yourself another cup of strong coffee.

After work you go home on time hoping to enjoy the evening with your spouse. They have not returned from work yet and you should probably pay the three overdue bills and insurance renewal waiting on your home desk, but it has been a hard day, so instead you pour yourself a glass of wine and flop down on the sofa to watch television. The news bulletin presents a world of economic crises, war and natural disasters, and the advert break reminds you of the expensive holiday you cannot afford. You awake to your spouse's amusement at you having dozed off in front of the television again.

Unless you work in a zoo, wild animals probably no longer pose a threat, but many modern-day activities cause the same fight-or-flight reaction that wolves caused our ancestors. But while our ancestors could release the stress by throwing a rock at the wolves or running, we are forced by societal pressures to behave. So all that adrenaline hangs around in our veins. This makes us edgy and we overreact to things. Then to escape the daily stress we look forward to weekends, where we seek to distract ourselves with drinking, extreme sports, sex or drugs.

In moderation, these things are good. However, many people take it too far and their efforts to relax have the opposite effect. If you have worked a stressful eighty-hour week, you probably need sleep more than you need a pub crawl, or to go bungee jumping. In excess, these things can increase stress by making us tired, depressed, and emotionally chaotic.

At other times we look forward to holidays, where we spend our free evenings researching the 'best' place, go on tours, eat, drink, and party too much, then fly home and get back to work before we have even had time to unpack. All this can be bad for our health.

How a Harvard researcher used a goose to discover the fight-or-flight response

Powdered rice was used as a primitive lie-detector test for thieves in India some 2,000 years ago. Suspects would be sat in a row and given a tablespoon of powdered rice each to chew. At the end of five minutes, they were ordered to spit the rice onto a fig leaf. The suspect whose rice was dry when he spat it out was deemed to be the thief. The rationale was that being nervous makes the mouth dry. The test was not perfect, because some thieves are good at lying, and some innocent people might get a nervous dry mouth when they are falsely accused. In spite of its imperfection, the idea behind this primitive test – that our nerves change when we are stressed out by lying – underpins the lie-detector tests we use today. The notion is that our bodies react automatically when we perceive a threat. A Harvard researcher called Walter

Cannon discovered the details of this automatic reaction more than a hundred years ago.

X-rays had just been discovered when Cannon graduated from medical school. At the time scientists argued about how food passed from the mouth to the stomach. Some scientists thought the act of swallowing pushed the food down the stomach with a single forced effort. Others thought it was massaged down slowly by wave-like contractions called peristalsis. In an effort to discover the truth, Cannon used X-rays to watch geese swallow buttons. He chose geese because their long necks provided more time to observe the process. (I don't know how he persuaded geese to swallow buttons.)

People did not realise how bad X-rays could be at that time, and there were not as many animal-rights activists around to stop him. Cannon defended the use of animals for his research and claimed to treat them very well. Using X-rays, he saw clearly the wave-like peristalsis in action, and the scientific debate was resolved. Next he showed that dogs and cats swallow in the same way as geese. He also observed signs of peristalsis in cats' and dogs' stomachs and digestive tracts. This led him to make a surprise discovery.

One day he was watching a cat digest food when dogs in a nearby room started barking loudly. This made the cats agitated, and in many cases halted the peristalsis in their stomachs and intestines. This seemed strange to him, so he contacted his friend, the famous Russian psychologist Ivan Pavlov, who was doing related experiments with dogs. Pavlov, famous for the 'Pavlov's Dog' experiments that I will talk about more in the upcoming chapter on conditioning, was happy to hear about Cannon's experiments because he had made a similar discovery. When Pavlov's dogs heard another dog barking aggressively, they would become excited and growl, and stop producing the gastric fluids required for digestion. Together, Pavlov and Cannon proved that when dogs and cats felt threatened, they stopped digesting.

During the First World War, Cannon was sent to the front

line to treat soldiers suffering from traumatic shock, where he made two more discoveries about the fight-or-flight response. First, humans react similarly to cats and dogs when they get scared. Not only does our digestion stop, but a host of other changes occur: our mouths get dry, our pupils dilate, our heart rates rise, and our adrenaline and cortisone levels rise. Basically, he discovered what happened to our caveman when he saw the wolf.

Second, Cannon discovered that the physiological changes that make up the fight-or-flight response come as a package, happening more or less simultaneously. He supposed that there must be a single 'switch' that activated all of these things. Eventually he called this group of nerves that get activated during the fight-or-flight response the 'sympathetic nervous system'. A nerve is like an electrical cable that sends information from one part of the body to another, for example from the brain to the stomach. The sympathetic nervous system is an interconnected set of nerves linking the brain and spinal cord to the parts of your body that you need to fight or run that I described above (such as the eyes, the adrenal glands, the leg and arm muscles, and so on).

A few years after Cannon's discoveries, a man called Hans Selye found that even small things can cause mini fight-or-flight responses.

Selye's bad news: we can't escape stress

Born in Vienna and raised in Hungary, Hans Selye began researching stress following his move to Montreal, Canada in 1936. He found that almost everything we do in life causes a mini fight-or-flight response that he called the 'stress response'. Most things in life cause stress, including illness, the excitement of our favourite sports team winning a game, or the upset of the same team losing a game. Whether we are worrying about our job or our finances, or feeling happy because we are getting a pay rise, we get a stress response.

We get the same reaction when falling in love or breaking up with a partner. Almost any new experience causes a mini stress response. Since every day brings new things, every day brings stress. Even if your days are all the same, worrying about your boredom can cause you stress.

Some scientists estimate that we have fifty stress responses per day, and a recent survey conducted by the American Psychological Association found that twenty-five per cent of Americans rated their stress levels at eight or more on a ten-point scale. The stress problem is getting worse, with stress levels rising ten per cent between 2012 and 2013 in the US. In fact, according to a US Surgeon General report in 1999, anxiety and stress-related disorders are the major contributors to mental illness in the US. Nobody knows for sure why stress is rising. It might be because jobs are less secure and most of the population in the developed nations are having more and more trouble paying their bills. It could be that the media bombards us constantly with bad news, or that traditional relationship roles are breaking apart, making family life more difficult. It is probably a combination of all of these.

On top of all this, it is getting more difficult to switch off. Our awesome mobile-phone technology means that our emails, messages and reminders follow most of us into bed. Perhaps counterintuitively, affluence is another cause of increased stress. Ready-made food at the supermarket means we do not have to chop food, let alone hunt. The easy availability of drugs from high-street pharmacies means we do not have to deal with headaches or colds. And health and safety laws mean children don't have to deal with adversity while they grow up. All this is great in many ways; however, since we are so protected, we have lost the ability to deal with challenges and stress.

Suspecting all this stress was bad, Selye looked for a cure. He worked tirelessly and ended up publishing forty books and 1,700 articles on the problem. Sadly for those seeking to banish stress from their lives, his main discovery was that stress cannot be avoided. The best we can do, according to Selye, is to manage it. Once a reporter challenged Selye, saying that he must be under a great deal of stress because he worked so hard. He admitted that he did work very hard, but he said he only engaged in activities he could 'win', that he could manage. Unfortunately, Selye did not explain how we can choose wisely to focus on activities that we, too, can win or manage.

I will explain some techniques to do just that in the next chapter. A better understanding of the strength of the links between stress and ill health might also motivate you to use them.

Stress and health: the damaging facts

Heart disease is caused when the heart's blood supply is blocked by a build-up of fatty substances in the blood vessels around the heart. This can lead to heart attacks and strokes. While it used to affect mostly older people, heart disease now affects a larger number of younger, working people. Today it is the leading cause of death in the world, killing over seven million people each year. We have known for a long time that obesity and lack of exercise can increase the risk of heart disease. Other psychological factors like depression, anxiety and financial stress can also increase the risks.

We have recently learned that stress is also an important contributor to heart disease. A group of researchers in Germany identified four high-quality studies that together involved over 2,500 patients measuring the effects of stress on people with heart disease. The people in these trials had already been diagnosed with heart disease; for example, they had already had a heart attack, but they were now well enough to return to work. Soon after they went back to work, the patients were asked about their stress. They were asked things like:

- Does your job require you to work very fast?
- Does your job require you to work very hard?
- Do you have enough time for all your work tasks?
- Do you have the possibility to decide for yourself what should be done in your work?

They were also asked to confirm whether they worked in a quiet and pleasant atmosphere, people at their workplaces got along, they felt supported at work, and whether they got along with their supervisors. Participants were then monitored for three years. Taken together, the studies concluded that people who reported having lots of stress at work were sixty-five per cent more likely to have suffered a cardiovascular disease event such as a heart attack or stroke than those who did not feel stressed at work.

In one of the studies, a Swedish one, about ten per cent of people in the studies with high levels of stress died from cardiac disease compared to only five per cent of the people with low job stress.

Other evidence also suggests that too much stress increases the risk of sleeping disorders, depression, anxiety, autoimmune diseases, asthma, constipation, diabetes, cold sores, infertility, pain, post-traumatic stress disorder, tooth problems, slower wound healing, and sexual dysfunction.

A problem is that the evidence linking stress with ill health suffers from the 'chicken-and-egg problem'. What came first: the bad health or the stress? If bad health causes higher stress, then it is obvious that people with more stress die younger, since the highly stressed people are also less healthy.

The only way to solve the chicken-and-egg problem would be to do a randomised trial. In theory, we could take lots of people and expose only half of them to stressful situations. This would tell us whether stressful situations were bad for health, but it would also be unethical to randomise people to do unhealthy things then watch them die. More importantly, there are other good reasons to believe that stress actually does cause bad health.

For one, the authors of the studies on the links between stress and heart disease were pretty smart and used statistical techniques to help solve the chicken-and-egg problem. They asked people not only about their stress levels, but also about their general health at the beginning of the study. They did the best they could to make sure the people with high stress in their studies were not less healthy to start with. Another reason I believe the evidence about stress and health does not suffer from the chicken-and-egg problem is the link between stress and the immune system.

Stress and the immune system

A group of researchers in the US and Canada identified 293 studies that looked at what happens to our immune system when we are under stress. All but a handful showed that chronic stress suppressed the immune system. This happened in numerous ways, most often by either reducing natural killer cell activity, or increasing inflammation. The immune system is complex and these studies are not perfect; however, they all point in the same direction: chronic stress suppresses and confuses the immune system.

It is actually a bit more complex than that, because your immune system gets a short boost during a fight-or-flight response so you can survive a wolf bite. But too many stress responses each day messes with the immune system's on/off switch, which can increase the risk of an autoimmune disease. An autoimmune disease is one caused by your immune system turning itself on when it shouldn't.

The best example is an allergic reaction. If you inhale harmful bacteria, it is good to sneeze and have a runny nose to get them out. But if you swallow or eat something that is not intrinsically bad, like pollen, there is no need to sneeze.

Sneezing because of an allergic reaction is basically an immune-system reaction gone wrong. Other autoimmune diseases include asthma and rheumatoid arthritis, as well as much more serious illnesses such as multiple sclerosis, Crohn's disease and lupus. There are no randomised trials I am aware of that show stress causes these diseases. However, as we will see in the next chapter, *lowering* stress can reduce the symptoms of some of these diseases.

So what do we do about it? There are basically three ways to react to stress: run, fight or manage it.

1. One way to run away is to become a monk and live in the Himalayas chanting 'Om' all day. If you do this you will not have car payments, mortgages, bosses, or relationships to stress you out. I have a lot of respect for monks, and we could all probably benefit by learning some life simplifying techniques from them. But a monk's life is not for most of us.

2. Fighting stress does not have to involve wolves and stones. When you wake up and see an email that needs to be dealt with, reply before breakfast. When a bad driver makes you swerve, shout at them and report them to the police. Complain to the manager when a waiter doesn't bring your food quickly enough. Argue and confront everyone and everything that causes stress. The problem with fighting stress is that you are probably not releasing it fully, the way the caveman was when he threw a stone. You are letting stressors control you. And you might end up dead or in jail. You certainly won't make many friends.

3. Between these two extremes lies managing stress. It is what Selye hinted at when he suggested only engaging in activities we can 'win', or have some control over. Another way to put that is to avoid getting overwhelmed by stress. Besides the techniques we will learn in the next chapter, the very knowledge that you have some control over whether you get a stress response helps.

The cause of stress is not always 'out there' – it can also come from within

Before I had dogs of my own, I could not tell the difference between friendly barking and barking that meant a dog wished to bite me. Dogs scared me, so if I saw one when I went running I would get a fight-or-flight response right away. I would feel my body tense up and if I couldn't easily avoid the dog, I got ready to fight and I tried to scare it off by shouting. That all changed when I got dogs of my own. I learned about dog body language, and the differences between happy and aggressive barks. Now I am happy when I see a dog. Most dogs are friendly. It was not the barking that had caused my previous fear, but my ignorance. More generally, neither dogs nor rain are stressful in themselves. Our inner reactions to them generate our stress responses.

We have some choice over the way we perceive things, including those that seem to be bad at first. Michael Jordan was probably the best basketball player of all time, but he was not selected for the varsity team in his sophomore year in high school and played for the junior varsity. Instead of interpreting that as a negative, he saw it as an opportunity. It made him work twice as hard as anyone else, which is what made him so successful as a professional. So getting dropped from the team was actually a good thing.

Joe Greenstein, also known as the Mighty Atom, was one of the world's first strong men. He was born with so many diseases that doctors predicted he would not live past five years old. His illnesses made him realise how precious every day was and he used that passion to succeed. Mahatma Gandhi failed to start a revolution in South Africa before his epic success in India. The 'failures' of Jordan, the Mighty Atom, or Gandhi were an opportunity to learn and improve. When things that seem bad happen to me, I like to think of the story of the poor Chinese farmer:

Once upon a time there was a poor Chinese farmer who had only a son and a horse and a small piece of land. One day, the horse escaped into the hills. The farmer's neighbours came to visit because they felt sorry for him: he lost his only horse! 'What bad luck!' they said.

The farmer replied, 'Bad luck? Good luck? Who knows?' A week later, the horse returned with a herd of wild horses from the hills. This time the neighbours congratulated the farmer on his good luck. Now he had a whole herd of horses: he was rich! But he replied, 'Bad luck? Good luck? Who knows?'

Then, when the farmer's son was attempting to tame one of the wild horses, he fell off its back and broke his leg. Everyone thought this was bad luck. His only son was injured! Not the farmer, who said, 'Bad luck? Good luck? Who knows?'

A few weeks later the army marched in to recruit all the young men to fight a war. Since the farmer's son had a broken leg, the army let him go.

'Bad luck? Good luck? Who knows?'

The fact that a more positive attitude towards life can help does not take away the fact that some things suck. When I told my colleague Sir Iain Chalmers about stress being (partly) under our control, he said, 'Tell my friends in Gaza whose houses are being bombed that stress is just in their minds.' Iain is right. It is ridiculous to suggest to starving people or those living in a war zone that their worries are just in their heads. I have never been in a war zone, and the closest I have come to starving is a voluntary fast.

Yet I can empathise a little bit with how these people might feel from the time when my mother suffered from metastatic breast cancer and was going through radical treatment. She was the most loving mother any child could have wanted. She was the closest thing to an angel I will ever know. She did not deserve to suffer. She tried everything from chemotherapy to diets to trying to gain weight (or lose weight), and

88

nothing worked, because the cancer was too aggressive. I really tried to help her relax, but the cancer and the radio-therapy had messed with her brain, so she even had trouble doing that. On top of that, she was worried about what would happen to her children once she was gone, even though we were all grown up. So I know that when things really suck, changing your mind does not change much.

That is why, if anyone is reading this book and something really terrible is happening, I am not telling you to snap out of it because it is only in your mind.

Fortunately, most of our problems are not that serious. It is much easier to adopt a positive attitude and reaction to things that suck less than fatal metastatic breast cancer, or living in a war zone. Ironically, one of the people who inspired this book is one of Iain's friends, Khamis Elessi, who does live in Gaza. I met Khamis when he came to Oxford to attend one of my courses. The day I met him he had completed a three-day ordeal just to arrive in the UK. His journey had involved multiple passport checks, full body searches, delayed planes and numerous other indignities. He was worrying about his family back at home. On top of all that, he knew it would be difficult for him to pass the course at Oxford because there was no good Internet access where he was staying. This made it almost impossible to complete the online activities that were required for the course.

Yet on the first morning of the course he arrived before all the other students with a big smile on his face. He turned out to be one of the happiest, friendliest and most bubbly people I have met. He participated actively and respectfully with other students from all walks of life and all religions, and with a wide variety of political beliefs in class discussions. After I drafted this story, I emailed him to ask if he was okay with me using his name and story in my book. His response was as inspiring as his story:

Dear Beloved Teacher,

I thank you so much for your kind message . . . smile is the most natural and spontaneous expression of happiness. The Secret of my Positivity and persistent smile most of the time is that I strongly believe in destiny meaning 'what will be will be' but at the same time we are gifted with a free and amazing power of healing wounds, building bridges of trust and beautifying our lives and that of others, which is the 'SMILE'. It takes less effort to show, fewer muscles to exhibit and shorter time to show its effect. It is an effective and instantaneous remedy for worries, distrust and disputes . . . It can bring back hope and light as the way forward for us. I always say 'whatever your brain can imagine, your hand will achieve one day'. There is no excuse for me and many others not to smile when we are being gifted and cared for by Great brothers, teachers and friends . . . Despite everything . . . Keep smiling.

With my highest respect,
Khamis

Khamis's positive attitude and smile do help him deal with his difficult circumstances in a more constructive way. If you watch the news, you might think that stories like Khamis's are rare, but they are not. You only have to look for them (and avoid most mainstream news). I recently found another inspiring story about a lady called Alice Herz-Sommer.

Alice was a renowned concert pianist who recently died at the age of 110. If you looked at the facts of her life, you would not be crazy for assuming that she might have been bitter. As a young woman during the Second World War she was taken to a concentration camp where her husband and most of her family died. She and her son survived, but her son later died prematurely of an aneurysm. In her old age, she lived alone for years in London in a single-room apartment and suffered a great deal of pain. Yet she never stopped playing the piano and never stopped moving, and never stopped being friendly to anyone who visited her.

How did she remain positive? In her words: 'I look at the good. When you are relaxed, your body is always relaxed. When you are pessimistic, your body behaves in an unnatural way. It is up to us whether we look at the good or the bad. When you are nice to others, they are nice to you. When you give, you receive.'

If circumstances in the world were the sole cause of stress, then Khamis Elessi and Alice Herz-Sommer should have been stressed and unhappy, but they weren't. And if things in the world made us relaxed and happy then people who had beauty, wealth and fame like Marilyn Monroe and Michael Jackson should have been blissful, but they were not. At least up to a point, the source of our stress is inside us.

Takeaways: Five easy things to move away from stress and anxiety

The most evidence-based ways to deal with stress are to relax and meditate, and we will talk about those in the next chapter. In the meantime, here are five things I use and that you might find helpful:

1. **Breathe to relax.** The easiest way to move from the fight-or-flight to the feed-and-breed response is to slow down your breathing. Randomised trials show that regulating the breath can reduce anxiety and stress. To do this simple exercise, breathe in for six seconds, and then breathe out for six seconds. If you can't look at a clock, then make your best guess at the timing. If six seconds is too long, then try five, or four seconds. Just breathe in as slowly as is comfortable, then breathe out as slowly as is comfortable. Try it now and see how you feel. Most people find that slowing the breath calms the mind and the body. I demonstrate this on my seven-minute YouTube video in a video called 'Slow Breath for Reducing Stress'.

2. **Take action.** Instead of worrying about stress, ask yourself, 'What concrete action can I take to address the thing that is causing me stress?' If your car breaks down, switch your attention from worrying to fixing it or calling a tow truck. If you can't think of a concrete action that will address the problem, *any* action will do. Do something altruistic (see Chapter Twelve). Go for a run. Jump up and down. Scream. Almost any action will help you feel better. If you are calm enough to sit down, you can read inspirational stories or do the 'what if' exercise.

3. **Inspirational stories.** Khamis's and Alice's stories are great for reducing worry and stress. Here are some more:

   - Hellen Keller (1880–1968) became deaf and blind before her second birthday. Despite this, she learned to read and write, and became the first deaf-blind person to gain a bachelor degree. She campaigned on issues of social welfare, women's suffrage, disability rights and impressed many with her force of personality.
   - Beethoven (1770–1827) became deaf. For a musician to lose his hearing is the greatest possible misfortune. Yet, despite the inevitable frustration, it did not stop Beethoven composing some of the most sublime pieces of music in history.
   - Rosa Parks (1913–2005) could have easily been just another statistic in the American system of racial segregation. In the Deep South, black Americans were systematically discriminated against, but on one famous day in 1955, Rosa Parks made a stand and refused to give up her seat to a white passenger. Her brave act of defiance sparked a widespread boycott of buses in Montgomery, Alabama, and inspired the modern civil-rights movement in the US.

A list of other inspirational stories can be found on this website: www.biographyonline.net/people/overcame-difficult-odds.html. If you are religious it might be a story from the Bible, Torah, Koran or the Bhagavad Gita.

4. **The 'what if' exercise.** Think of the thing that is making you feel stressed. It might be that you are having trouble following a diet, you want a better job or a great relationship. If nothing specific comes to mind, it could be stress itself. Then ask yourself the 'what if' question. Here are some I am asking or have asked in the past:

> What if I was following the diet properly?
> What if I had my dream job?
> What if I had that amazing relationship?
> What if I could revolutionise and improve the way people view their bodies and their health?

Close your eyes and imagine what it would feel like if all those 'ifs' came true. Try to imagine through all your senses, and in as much detail as possible.

For example: how would you feel if you followed that diet? What would you say? How would you look? How would the world look? How would you and the world be if you had that dream job, to have that peaceful loving relationship . . . ? How will you use the 'new and improved' you to help the world?

Write this down.

Then leave it for an hour while you have lunch, dinner, a bath or a break. Then read it quietly. Read it aloud if you like. Read it as often as you like. The best time is when you first wake up or just before you go to bed. This will help you have a new attitude towards any potential worries.

5. **Don't add stress to your stress.** It is one thing to worry about something (maybe your car broke down). Then you might realise you are stressed and after reading this chapter you might say to yourself, 'Oh no, I'm stressed and that is bad for my health!' If you do that you are worrying about two things: your car broke down, and you are

stressed about being stressed. Focus on a solution to the problem (your car breaking down), and ignore being stressed about being stressed. It doesn't help and it does not make sense.

6

How a Yogi Taught the Beatles to Relax

*Don't worry about the future. Or worry, but know that
worrying is as effective as trying to solve an algebra equa-
tion by chewing bubble gum.*

Mary Schmich, American journalist
and Pulitzer Prize winner

India's Maharishi Mahesh Yogi takes on Harvard's Herbert Benson

In 1967, doctor and cardiologist Herbert Benson was doing
blood-pressure experiments with monkeys at Harvard Medical
School. That was also the year that the Beatles started looking
for meaning in their lives. In Paul McCartney's words: 'We'd
been into drugs, the next step is . . . to try and find a meaning.'
So when an Indian guru called Maharishi Mahesh Yogi visited
London, the Beatles visited him. They liked what he said, so
in 1968 the band members took their wives and girlfriends
to India to do a meditation retreat with him. Inevitably, an
army of newspaper and television reporters followed. When
the media arrived there, they found even more stars at the
Maharishi's Ashram: Mike Love from the Beach Boys, Mia
Farrow, and Donovan were already there. Although the
Maharishi did his best to give the stars some peace by keeping
the reporters away, their visit was publicised all over the
world. Eastern spirituality suddenly became very trendy.

Emboldened by the Maharishi's fame, some of his meditators
visited Harvard researcher Herbert Benson. They told him that
the kind of meditation the Maharishi taught, called transcendental meditation, could reduce blood pressure the same way
that drugs could. Initially Benson thought this was too wacky
and politely sent them away. But the meditators were persistent

95

and kept coming back. Eventually Benson decided to get rid of them by doing a proper trial of transcendental meditation to prove once and for all that it did not work. Benson also had a condition: he would only study meditation if the Maharishi Yogi himself agreed to participate. That way, when Benson proved the technique didn't work, he would expose the Maharishi as a charlatan. For his part, the Maharishi was convinced that meditation did work, so he agreed to Benson's condition. He looked forward to a Harvard researcher giving the practice a firm scientific basis.

Benson set up the experiment by connecting meditators to mouthpieces, nose clips and tight-fitting facemasks. These conditions were not conducive to deep relaxation. In spite of this, Benson's first study with thirty-six meditators aged seventeen to forty-one years old found that meditation lowered breathing rates, oxygen consumption, and blood acidity (which is associated with stress). The first study did not show a change in blood pressure, but that was because the meditators were young, healthy, and already had low blood pressure. He did a follow-up study with older patients who had high blood pressure and found that meditation lowered blood pressure by a similar amount as drugs.

Benson described the state induced by meditation as a 'wakeful hypermetabolic physiologic state'. It was similar to sleep, because the inner conditions for regeneration and recovery were being induced. But the meditators were not actually asleep, and the brain-wave frequencies observed during meditation were those associated with deep relaxation, rather than the frequencies observed during deep sleep. It was basically the opposite of the fight-or-flight response described in the last chapter.

Whereas the fight-or-flight response is associated with the sympathetic nervous system, the relaxation response involves the *parasympathetic* nervous system. The word 'para' in Greek means 'against' or 'contrary to'. That's why a nickname for the effects produced by the sympathetic nervous system is the 'fight-or-flight' response, and the effect produced by the para-sympathetic system is called the 'feed-and-breed' response. The parasympathetic nervous system is composed of the linked nerves connecting your brain and spinal cord to numerous organs of your body to help you to relax, digest and breed. Parasympathetic nerves activate the body's digestive system, the sexual organs, and other nerves responsible for slowing down the heart and breathing rate. When there is no need to fight or run, we can relax, enjoy our food, and think about other more pleasant things. That is when the parasympathetic nervous system is active.

There are three main ways that relaxation and meditation activate the feed-and-breed (parasympathetic nervous system) response. First, relaxation and meditation take your mind away from the mental sources of stress, and we saw in the last chapter that a lot of the sources of stress come from our minds rather than the outside world itself. When you are focusing on your body or your breath, your mind is not preoccupied with what your work colleague did to you yesterday, or how you plan to take revenge tomorrow. With the mind no longer focused on the source of the stress, your body and mind can relax.

Second, when you relax, your breathing rate slows down. Since the parasympathetic system comes as a whole (as you know if you did last chapter's exercise, and I will explain more about this immediately below), the slower breathing rate activates *everything* associated with the parasympathetic nervous system. So you get a full 'feed-and-breed' response, just by slowing the breath.

Finally, in meditation (and, obviously, the relaxation response) your body is more relaxed. Allowing your *body* to relax sends a message to your brain that things are okay, that there is no threat, and that you can move into the feed and breed reponse. So the parasympathetic system counteracts the sympathetic nervous system. Even though the sympathetic and parasympathetic nervous systems are opposites in many ways, they share two important qualities.

- Both systems come more or less as whole packages that get switched on or off together. If you see a wolf, it is not just your pupils that dilate: all the other things like increased heart rate, suppressed digestion, and lung vessel dilation happen together. Similarly, the body muscles seem to relax in a connected way. There is some evidence that if you relax your jaw, your whole body relaxes.

- They are both part of the body's *autonomic* (a fancy word for 'automatic') nervous system, meaning they are usually not within our conscious control. When your brain perceives a wolf, the fight-or-flight response kicks in without you telling it to do so. When you lie down tired after a long day, your relaxation response kicks in in a similarly automatic way. Contrast this with the part of the nervous system that is within our conscious control. When I move my fingers to type these words, or when I reach for my tea, my hands are consciously directed by my will. Philosophers debate the possibility of free will, but we will leave that for another day.

  There is one thing to add about the automatic nature of the sympathetic and parasympathetic systems. They are not completely automatic because, as we saw in the take-away from the last chapter, and as we will see from the takeaways in this chapter, we have some control over them. The easiest way to influence them is by consciously regulating our breathing.

Benson wanted to publish what he found out about meditation for the scientific community around the world. But he had a problem. Just as he was sure that transcendental meditation was bunk until he saw it work with his own eyes, his Harvard colleagues were likely to think the same thing. They might think Benson was becoming an alternative long-haired hippie, who had started smoking too much marijuana with the Beatles. But Benson was smart and he thought of a way to share his discoveries with the world without being viewed as a quack.

His trick was instead of using the term 'transcendental meditation', he used 'relaxation'. He wrote a book called *The Relaxation Response* that quickly became a bestseller. Benson's use of a new name did not only help him avoid getting ostracised by his colleagues. It was also more accurate. The Maharishi's transcendental meditation was great, but it is not the only game in town. There are hundreds if not thousands of types of meditation out there. I have tried about thirty different kinds myself.

Besides meditation, hypnosis, some kinds of prayer, and traditional yoga all have similar physiological effects as the relaxation response. By traditional yoga, I mean forms that involves breathing techniques and mindfulness alongside the poses. (Most yoga practised in the West focuses mostly on the poses and physical benefits.) The relaxation response is common to all of these practices, so Benson did more than choose a new name, he found that many of these practices share a common effect: they all activate the parasympathetic nervous system and the relaxation response.

More recently, 'mindfulness' has become all the rage. You can do courses in it, download apps to help you develop it, and Harvard Business School teaches you how to use mindfulness to be a more effective leader. The mainstream use of the word mindfulness has its origins in a similar re-branding to the one Benson pulled off when he dropped the word 'transcendental meditation' in favour of the 'relaxation response'. Here's what happened.

The godfathers of mindfulness such as Jon Kabat-Zinn started off as Buddhist meditators and they faced the same problems with their families that Benson experienced with his colleagues. Their non-Buddhist Christian or Jewish family members thought Buddhism was incompatible with their religions, despite its lack of a God to worship. So Kabat-Zinn began using the word 'mindfulness' in place of 'Buddhist meditation'. He also took away all the foreign words and rituals like chanting. As a result, Christians, Jews and Muslims can practise Buddhist meditation without offending their priests, rabbis and mullahs, as long as they call it mindfulness.

Anyone who has experienced and understands the rudiments of Buddhist meditation and mindfulness will tell you that the two practices are very similar. Sometimes they look very different, because mindfulness teachers often teach in jeans and have normal hairstyles, whereas most Buddhist monks shave their heads and wear robes. And there is often some chanting before a Buddhist meditation session. All the chanting I have heard simply involves repetition of simple, non-religious phrases like 'please give me inner peace'. It does not refer to any God.

Also you can do the meditation without doing the chanting. More important than the difference between Buddhist meditation and mindfulness is the difference between individual teachers. It is important to find a teacher who is qualified, and who you feel comfortable with. Strange questions can arise when we sit still for a while and have a good teacher to debrief with can help. The choice of an appropriate teacher is an individual one. A teacher who is great for me might not suit you and vice versa.

Because the word mindfulness avoids spooking people, and because it helps most people, it has spread like wildfire. In the end, it doesn't matter what word you use and it does not matter whether you prefer relaxation, traditional yoga or something else. If you are interested in it, the important thing is that you do it, because it can improve your health.

Evidence that the relaxation response improves health

A recent systematic review that contained four randomised trials involving a total of 430 participants showed that practising the Maharishi's transcendental meditation for fifteen to twenty minutes, twice per day, could lower blood pressure and help people live longer. One of these trials found that three years after it had ended, all of the participants who meditated were still alive, compared to only seventy-seven per cent of those who did not, meaning that meditation seemed to increase survival by twenty-three per cent. The trials in the review were small, so more studies are needed to investigate the benefits of meditation. However, when considered alongside studies of similar techniques such as yoga and Tai Chi, we see similar benefits, making the transcendental meditation results quite credible.

It can also reduce anxiety and depression. A large review including forty-seven randomised trials involving a total of 3,515 people found that mindfulness had similar effects as drugs for reducing stress, anxiety, pain and depression by over ten per cent, which is roughly the same or better as many common drugs for these ailments, but without the side effects. The practice was also shown to improve quality of life. One trial in the review looked at people who had the challenging task of caring for a family member with dementia. It can be dangerous to leave people with dementia alone, so the carers cannot leave them alone. This causes carers to neglect their hobbies, exercise and friends.

It is often a stressful role, so it should not surprise us that people who care for family members with dementia develop numerous health problems of their own as a result. In the study, half of a group of seventy-eight caregivers were given a mindfulness training course, while the other half were given additional education and support. After six months, the group that did mindfulness had twenty-five-per-cent less stress than the group that just had simple education. There was no change in anxiety, but depression was reduced by ten-per-cent more in the mindfulness group. These effects are bigger than the effects of drugs for stress and depression reduction.

The number of systematic reviews in this area is growing and almost universally positive, showing that these techniques are sometimes as good as many common drugs, or can be used alongside the drugs to enhance outcomes. The other great thing is that none of the studies show any significant harmful side effects. Here is a sample of diseases that systematic reviews show relaxation can help cure:

- **Anxiety and stress.** Two systematic reviews with a total of seventy-four trials and over 5,000 patients showed that relaxation therapy/mindfulness reduces anxiety by over ten per cent.
- **Arthritis.** A systematic review of eleven randomised trials showed mindfulness therapy reduces chronic pain such as arthritis.
- **Asthma.** One review with fifteen trials suggests that relaxation techniques improve lung function in asthmatic patients. A more recent randomised trial showed mindfulness improves quality of life and reduces stress in those with asthma, and another found that relaxation techniques could reduce blood pressure in pregnant women with bronchial asthma.
- **Depression.** A review including twelve randomised trials suggests a modest benefit of relaxation meditation for reducing depressive symptoms. Another review with six randomised trials suggests mindfulness can prevent relapse into depression.
- **Diabetes mellitus.** A review with four trials found that yoga is likely to improve diabetic symptoms in patients with Type II diabetes. Another review with five trials found it has positive short-term benefits on fasting blood glucose levels.
- **Hypertension (high blood pressure).** A review of 107 studies shows meditation reduces high blood pressure.
- **Insomnia.** A review with 112 studies suggests that most trials of mind/body techniques reduce insomnia symptoms.
- **Irritable bowel syndrome (IBS).** A review of eight trials found that relaxation meditation can reduce IBS symptoms.
- **Low back pain.** A review including ten randomised controlled trials involving a total of 967 patients found

strong evidence for short-term effectiveness and moderate evidence for long-term effectiveness of yoga in reducing chronic low back pain.

- **Multiple sclerosis.** A review with four high-quality randomised trials showed that mind-body interventions including yoga, mindfulness, relaxation and biofeedback (a technique whereby people monitor bodily parameters such as heart rate in order to learn to control them) reduced a variety of multiple sclerosis symptoms.
- **Psychological health (wellbeing) of cancer patients.** A review of three randomised trials of an intervention that combines mindfulness with yoga reported positive results, including improvements in mood, sleep quality and reductions in stress, which can help improve subjective wellbeing (including reducing depression and anxiety symptoms) and quality of life.
- **Stress due to HIV/AIDS.** A review of six trials show that the relaxation response or traditional meditation/mindfulness can help improve the following health problems that HIV patients often suffer from: anxiety and stress, asthma, arthritis, depression, diabetes mellitus, hypertension (high blood pressure), insomnia, irritable bowel syndrome, low back pain, multiple sclerosis symptoms, and wellbeing.

Some studies also show the relaxation response can boost the immune system. There is even evidence that relaxing helps you solve problems.

Relaxation and creativity

Besides health benefits, the relaxation response can also help us think of creative solutions to problems, including solutions to things that cause stress. Let me explain with the candle problem. A candle, matches and a small box of drawing pins are all lying on a table. The table is up against the wall, and there is a corkboard on the wall. Your task is to fix the candle onto the corkboard in such a way that the wax does not drip on the table below. If you have never tried this riddle, stop reading here and have a go (or think about how you might solve the problem).

Duncker's (1945) Candle Problem

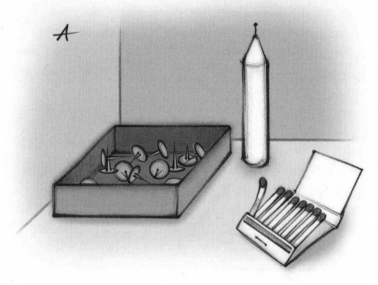

The subjects are asked to attach a candle to the wall and are given a box of tacks, candles, and matches as shown in panel A. The solution is shown in panel B.

People often try attaching the candle to the corkboard with drawing pins, but that does not work because the pins are not long enough to go through the candle. Others try to melt the candle wax on the side of the candle then stick it to the wall. But that doesn't work because the corkboard is too slippery and the candle falls. Eventually many people figure out that the solution is to empty the drawing pins from the box, pin the box to the corkboard, place the candle in the box and then light it.

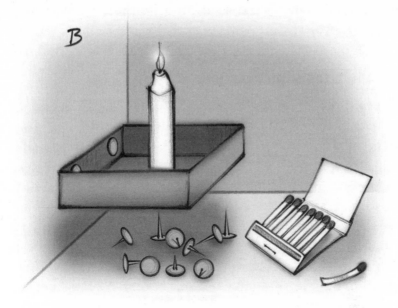

In 1962 Sam Glucksberg modified the problem by offering a reward. He told some of the subjects: 'Depending on how quickly you solve the problem you can win five dollars or twenty dollars. The fastest twenty-five per cent of the subjects in your group will win five dollars; the fastest individual will receive twenty dollars.'

Adjusting for inflation, the amounts in today's dollars would be approximately forty dollars and 150 dollars. Now you might think that the reward made people solve the problem faster because they would win money. In fact, the opposite happened. People who were offered a reward performed *worse* than the subjects who were not offered a reward. How can we explain this? It turned out the process of turning the task into a competition can create stress in subjects, which can activate the stress response. Stress is good for running away from a wolf, but it undermines the ability to solve creative problems. This makes perfect sense: if a wolf is chasing you it's the wrong time to think about poetry or creative projects.

How the relaxation response works

In a word, the relaxation response (and techniques that activate it such as meditation, traditional yoga, Tai Chi, etc.) activates the parasympathetic nervous system. This includes the digestive system and the immune system. Studies measure immune system markers like inflammatory proteins, immune cell count and antibody response. Their results confirm mindfulness meditation can positively affect all of these by allowing the immune system to do its job better. The relaxation response also improves our ability to digest and absorb the nutrients we need to nourish and replenish our bodies. All this happens automatically when we just relax. But we do have some conscious control over the relaxation response.

Change your mind to relax more

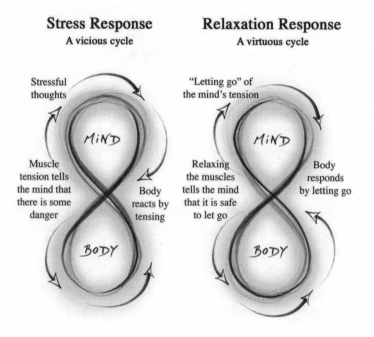

Stress Response
A vicious cycle

Stressful thoughts

MiND

Muscle tension tells the mind that there is some danger

Body reacts by tensing

BODY

Relaxation Response
A virtuous cycle

"Letting go" of the mind's tension

MiND

Relaxing the muscles tells the mind that it is safe to let go

Body responds by letting go

BODY

A simple but interesting study carried out by Abiola Keller and colleagues at the University of Wisconsin suggests that having a relaxed attitude towards stress can *reverse* the harms that stress induces. The group examined the responses of almost 30,000 Americans to two questions from a previous study. These were:

1. During the past twelve months, would you say that you experienced a lot of stress, a moderate amount of stress, relatively little stress, or almost no stress at all?
2. During the past twelve months, how much effect has stress had on your health – a lot, some, hardly any, or none?

The people who answered 'a lot' to the first question were more likely to have poor health outcomes. These people said they had a lot of stress and they were forty-three per cent more likely to die relative to the group who were not worried about stress. This is expected, given what we know about the stress response and its negative effects on the immune and other systems.

The surprise came when the researchers looked at people who answered 'hardly any' or 'none' to the second question. This group, which included people who said they had experienced a lot of stress, did not think stress was bad for their health and so were not worried about it. These participants had better health outcomes even than those who reported having very little stress. Being an observational study, we face the chicken-and-egg problem again: did not worrying about stress lead to better health? Or did better health make people worry less about stress? And if you are not worried about stress, are you actually stressed? We cannot be sure what the answers to these questions are.

In her TED talk, health psychologist Kelly McGonigal does not refer to the chicken-and-egg problem with observational studies and claims that worrying about stress, rather than stress itself, is the fifteenth leading cause of death in the United States. The main study she uses to justify this claim is not definitive, but her main message that we should stop worrying is a good one, because we have some control over it. Worrying rarely helps and almost always increases our stress levels. So it is important to take time every day to relax.

Takeaway: Inducing the relaxation response

One way to learn to relax is to follow in the Beatles' footsteps and visit an Ashram in India, but you don't have to. There are many options, including meditation, mindfulness, traditional yoga, Tai Chi, Qi Kong, and Benson's method. I will describe an exercise I teach that is evidence-based. All you really need is about fifteen minutes and a quiet space where it is safe to close your eyes. It is quite easy and will make you feel good right away.

Conscious relaxation

This is how I do and teach relaxation. It is also informed by my knowledge of the evidence for yoga. It is best to do this exercise lying down, but you can also do it seated. Take a few deep breaths or sighs (see previous exercises) and feel the tension in your body begin to let go. Prepare to squeeze and release muscles in different parts of your body. It is best to do this with your eyes closed, so read through it once then do it, or visit my YouTube channel to listen to one of the videos I've made.

- **Legs.** Bring your attention to your legs. Take a deep breath in, and squeeze all your leg muscles. Hold your breath as you squeeze your thighs, hamstrings, calves – all the leg muscles. Keep the other parts of your body completely relaxed as you squeeze your leg muscles. After a few seconds, suddenly release your breath with a sigh and simultaneously release all the tension in your leg muscles.
- **Arms.** Next, bring your attention to your arms. Breathe in, then hold your breath as you squeeze your fists and tighten all the muscles in your arms: your biceps, triceps and forearms. Keep the other parts of your body completely

relaxed as you squeeze your leg muscles. Then release your breath with a sigh and simultaneously release all the tension in your arm muscles.

- **Lower back.** Then, bring your attention to your lower back. Breathe in then hold your breath as you squeeze and tighten all the muscles in your lower back and your buttocks. If you feel strong you can lift your hips off the floor. Keep the other parts of your body completely relaxed as you squeeze your lower back and buttocks. Then release your breath with a sigh and simultaneously release all the tension in your lower back and buttocks. Drop your lower back to the ground.
- **Shoulders.** Now, bring your attention to your shoulders. Lift your shoulders up to your ears. Then push them as far away from your ears as you can. Then wiggle your shoulders around any way you want. Massage them into the ground. Feel all the tension from your shoulders and shoulder blades being released. Then take a deep breath in and sigh as you release the breath and relax the shoulders.
- **Neck.** As you inhale, slowly turn your head to the left, keeping your whole body relaxed other than the muscles in the neck. You may feel the upper vertebrae in your back twisting. Hold it there for one more long breath, then as you exhale slowly move your head to the centre, feeling all the tension in the neck release. Now repeat on the other side. As you inhale, slowly turn your head to the right . . .
- **Face and head.** Moving your attention to your face and head, close your eyes, take a deep breath in, and squeeze all the muscles in your face. Squeeze your eyes together, squeeze your jaw. As if you are trying to move everything on your face towards the tip of your nose. Hold your breath for a few seconds. Then sigh out the breath and suddenly relax all the muscles in your face. Feel all the tension melt away. Feel your jaw relax, feel your lips relax, feel your eyes relax, feel your eyebrows relax, and feel your forehead relax. Feel your entire scalp relax.

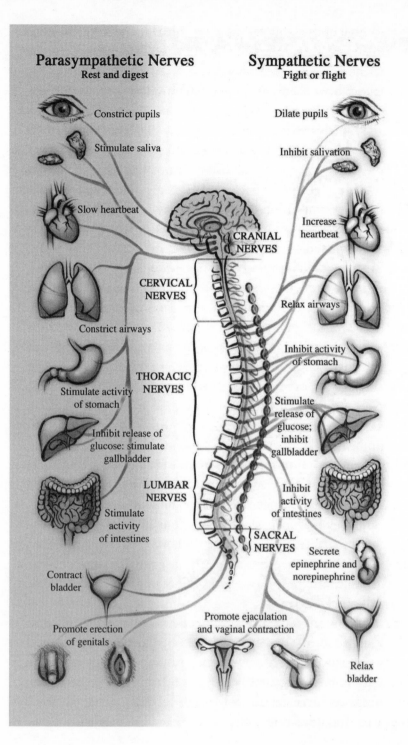

Parasympathetic Nerves
Rest and digest

Constrict pupils
Stimulate saliva
Slow heartbeat
Constrict airways
Stimulate activity of stomach
Inhibit release of glucose: stimulate gallbladder
Stimulate activity of intestines
Contract bladder
Promote erection of genitals

Sympathetic Nerves
Fight or flight

Dilate pupils
Inhibit salivation
Increase heartbeat
Relax airways
Inhibit activity of stomach
Stimulate release of glucose; inhibit gallbladder
Inhibit activity of intestines
Secrete epinephrine and norepinephrine
Promote ejaculation and vaginal contraction
Relax bladder

CRANIAL NERVES
CERVICAL NERVES
THORACIC NERVES
LUMBAR NERVES
SACRAL NERVES

- **Whole body**. Now feel all your muscles and all your bones relaxing. Feel your body heavy, sinking into the floor or chair. Let your breathing relax. There is no need to worry about how deeply you relax, or how to relax more deeply. Simply enjoy any level of relaxation you are experiencing. Stay in this space for between one and ten more minutes, depending on how much time you have.

Eustress and the zone

There is just one thing to add about the relaxation response: if we were totally relaxed all the time, we might not get out of bed. We need some stress to get things done. The problem is that most of us go too far and waste too much energy by getting much more stressed out than we have to. We need to regulate how much energy we use to minimise any damage done by stress, and we need to relax after our tasks so that stress does not linger on unnecessarily.

During my first few years as a rower, I used to get so nervous before races that I was tired during the actual races themselves. Without knowing it, I was putting my body into the same state as the mythical caveman I described at the beginning of the last chapter. Later I learned some simple relaxation techniques that helped me conserve my energy before the race. On very rare occasions, however, I was not nervous enough before a race, perhaps because I was tired or simply having a bad day. On these days, I had to learn techniques to lift my spirits. To perform well you have to get in the 'zone'.

The zone was first described by Robert M. Yerkes and John Dillingham Dodson in 1908. They realised that to do important tasks some stress is required, but not too much. The Yerkes-Dodson Law states that increased stress can raise your performance up to a point (this is eustress), after which it becomes counterproductive. Once we understand this, we can do things to increase our energy and stress levels or decrease them to make sure we stay in the zone.

Yerkes-Dodson Law

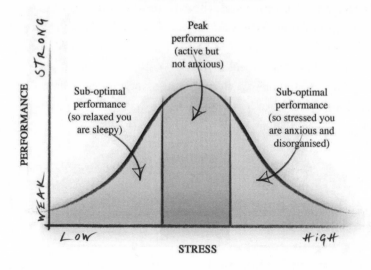

When I talk to people about the zone, there is always one person in the audience who insists that lots of stress is very good for them because it helps them get things done. Other than situations analogous to fighting a wolf, I cannot think of any circumstances in which 'beyond the zone' stress helps. And given the negative effect that being too stressed out has on health, even if it were true that having lots of stress was good, it would only be beneficial in the short term.

In fact, many people who look relaxed are escaping from the various things they need to do. What might come across as outwardly lazy behaviour can sometimes be exhaustion caused by busyness and stress. Of the thousands of people I have met in the twelve countries where I have lived, only one was totally relaxed.

He was a lovely Balinese man called Wayan, who was the main employee of a small hotel I stayed in for a week in a remote area of Bali. He would lie around in his hammock for most of the day. I think I saw him sweep the floor once very slowly. Whenever I told him I was ready for breakfast which was included in the rate, he would smile, say yes, and remain in his hammock for a few more minutes before walking slowly into the kitchen. He would emerge an hour or so later with toast and some fruit. One hour to make some toast! If he was any more relaxed, he might have starved to death. Wayan might have benefited from a bit more stress. Most of us are not like Wayan and could probably benefit from techniques that help us relax.

We have to know how to relax and how to get 'into the zone', but not beyond it.

Takeaway: Getting into the zone

There are many tools that can help you get 'into the zone' or in a state of 'flow', and a lot has been written about how you can become an expert at this. The two I will share here are very simple, and while they are not enough to induce your peak performance, they can help a great deal. The first one is to make you less stressed if you are feeling too anxious (this is the one that is usually needed), and the second one is to get you ready if you feel sleepy and not stimulated enough.

1. **Reducing stress if you are too anxious.** The best way to do this is with breathing exercises. See the slow breathing exercise from Chapter Four. If you feel too anxious you can do this, and your anxiety will reduce. Do it until you feel like you are back in the zone. Another easy breathing exercise is to sigh. Take a deep breath in, then hold the breath for as long as is comfortable. Then release the breath with a deep sighing sound.

2. **Giving yourself a kick-start if you are not anxious enough.** For me this is rare, but it happens sometimes. Again, an easy way to pick up your energy levels to get you in the zone is with the breath. But this time, instead of slowing down the breath, breathe in and out deeply a few times. You may need to do it more than three times to feel your energy levels rise. If you do too many, you may feel light-headed, so start with just a few.

7
It Is Never Just in Your Mind

Age is a question of mind over matter. If you don't mind,
it doesn't matter.

Satchel Paige, legendary
African-American baseball player

How Bruce Moseley got into placebos

Bruce Moseley is the team surgeon for the Houston Rockets
basketball team and he performs a lot of knee surgeries on
players. Arthroscopy is a common surgical procedure used
to examine and treat knee joints. To perform these surgeries,
Dr Moseley inserts a small metal tube called an arthroscope
into the knee and then uses it to repair damaged cartilage
and remove loose bone fragments that cause pain. A million
knee arthroscopies are performed each year in the US at
a cost of $5,000 each, making a total annual bill of $5 billion.

By observing that players with positive attitudes seemed to
recover more quickly, Dr Moseley got the idea that *placebo*
arthroscopy might be almost as good as the real thing. So he
found 180 patients who had such bad knee pain that even
the best drugs had failed to work for over six months. Many
were in so much pain they had trouble getting out of their
chairs. He gave half of them real arthroscopy and the other
half placebo arthroscopy. Patients in the placebo arthroscopy
group were given anaesthetics and a small incision was made
in their knees, but there was no arthroscope, no repairing of
damaged cartilage, and no cleaning out of loose fragments of
bone. To keep the patients ignorant about which group they
were in, the doctors and nurses talked through a real procedure even if they were performing the placebo procedure.

Bruce Moseley and his team then monitored the patients,

asking them how much pain they felt, and measured how far they could walk and how many stairs they could climb before their pain got in the way. After two years, even Bruce Moseley was surprised. The placebo was not almost as good as the real surgery, it was equally as good.

When I read Bruce Moseley's study, I was surprised because I had never heard of placebo surgery. And in spite of my research, I was sceptical about how surgery could cure what appeared to be a purely local, mechanical problem. I even wondered whether the people in the trial would have recovered without *any* surgery (placebo surgery or real surgery). Like the POWs in Cochrane's story from Chapter One, perhaps Moseley's patients were merely outstanding examples of how humans can get better without any treatment. However, this was not likely. The patients in the trial had not responded to even the best drugs for over six months. So the sham surgery seemed to have done something rather dramatic to these patients.

My next reaction was that the placebo surgery might have worked for subjective psychological issues such as feeling better, but not for more objective, physical outcomes. But the patients in the placebo group were able to climb more stairs and walk further than they were before, too. So the placebo surgery was effective for physical outcomes as well as psychological ones. I was still not convinced: how could a placebo fix a mechanical problem with the knee? So I thought maybe Moseley's study was a fluke. It wasn't. It turns out there have been other placebo surgery trials with comparable results.

Placebo back surgery

Vertebroplasty is a fancy name for making a small cut in someone's back then injecting bone cement (a kind of glue) into a damaged vertebra. In 2003, 25,000 Americans underwent this procedure. The number of people getting vertebroplasties is closer to 100,000 now, and they cost $5,000 each. So close to $500 million dollars are spent on vertebroplasty every year in the US alone.

Researchers from Australia took seventy-eight patients with spinal fractures. Half of them got the real thing, while the other half got fake vertebroplasty. To perform the placebo surgery, surgeons cut the skin and tapped the bone, but did not inject any cement. Patients didn't know whether they were getting the real or fake surgery. Patients who got the placebo procedure did as well as patients given the real procedure. In some ways the real vertebroplasty was worse, because patients who got it were more likely to need drugs. Not only that, the cement used to glue the fractured bone together often leaks, possibly causing more fractures, trouble controlling urination, and weakness in the legs.

Placebo arthroscopy and placebo vertebroplasty are not the only fake surgeries that work. Some of my colleagues at Oxford University recently researched over fifty placebo-controlled trials of various surgical techniques and they found that the placebo surgery was as good as the real surgery in more than half the trials.

I have been offered both back and knee surgery and I am happy that I have refused both. When I injured my back rowing, a surgeon proposed to operate on me but I was scared of the risks and refused. Some activities like heavy squats or cleans can still give me some back pain, but overall I have cured myself with yoga. Two years ago, I twisted my knee playing volleyball, and soon after (in spite of the pain) I ran a half-marathon. It hurt a lot during the run and the pain did not go away even after a few weeks of rest. I couldn't bend it more than forty-five degrees, and walking more than a few minutes hurt, so I had a scan.

The doctors told me my meniscus was chipped and I should get surgery. I thought it would be hypocritical to do the surgery since I was writing this book, so I chose physiotherapy instead. There is a lot of evidence that physiotherapy is great for reducing knee pain.

My knee is now almost completely better. I can almost bend it fully and I went for a three-hour run last week and it didn't bother me. I am not saying I will never have surgery, but if there is a more conservative, cheaper and less risky option, I will try that one first.

How does placebo surgery work?

Placebo surgery is likely to work via more than one mechanism. First placebo surgery activates systems that produce pain relieving drugs like endorphins and dopamine. As for the placebo knee surgery, I suspect that the star status of Bruce Moseley himself might have played a role, too. He is quite a character. How would you feel if you entered the operating room to see the guy you saw on the TV whenever you watched basketball?

One of the patients who got the placebo surgery was called Sylvester Colligan, who was seventy-six years old at the time. He was interviewed after they told him he had the placebo surgery. About Dr Moseley he said: 'I was very impressed with him, especially when I heard he was the team doctor with the [Houston] Rockets . . . So, sure, I went ahead and signed up for this new thing he was doing . . . The surgery was two years ago and the knee never has bothered me since . . . It is just like my other knee now. I give a whole lot of credit to Dr Moseley. Whenever I see him on the TV during a basketball game, I call the wife in and say, "Hey, there's the doctor that fixed my knee!"'

International placebo expert Dan Moerman met Dr Moseley and reports: 'He is a very impressive man. He's tall, strong and athletic looking. He has a firm, friendly and persuasive manner . . . he sure looks like a good surgeon to me, even though I've never seen him on TV, and I'm not much of a basketball fan.'

All this means that when Bruce Moseley treats you, you *expect* to get better. We will further explore how positive expectations can induce your body to produce its own pain-killers in Chapter Eight and how doctors with a good bedside manner can have a healing effect in Chapter Ten.

There is another explanation for how placebo surgery might work: it activates the body's power of regeneration called the 'wound-healing cascade'. All living organisms are very good at regenerating themselves when they get cut or injured. If you cut off an earthworm's head, it completely grows back. You can't grow a human head back if it gets chopped off, but your body can repair itself very well.

The wound-healing cascade is activated whenever you get a cut. The body does not know whether the cut is from a thorn that scrapes you or from a friendly surgeon's knife. It simply starts healing in the region where damage has occurred, even if the damage is caused by a friendly surgeon who is trying to help. It begins with blood clotting in the injured region to stop the bleeding. Then white blood cells 'phagocytose' unwanted cells. This is a fancy way of saying they eat them. Next the body makes new blood vessels in the region so that it can send more nutrients and growth hormones to rebuild the damaged area. Then, the wound is healed when new scar tissue and skin cover the wound.

Placebo back-pain surgery has an additional mechanism. When you get the placebo surgery, you are given a pretty hefty dose of local painkiller. This can cause your back pain to subside for some time. With less pain, you feel freer to move around, and the moving around might have a benefit (exercise reduces back pain).

Effective placebo surgery shows that more invasive and more expensive real surgery is less necessary than we think. It also suggests that positive beliefs about the outcome of a treatment can cure mechanical as well as psychological problems. I know a lot of people who have had knee and back surgery. Many of them need to return for further surgeries, and they rarely accept that there might have been a better option.

For instance, when I told someone I met at a Christmas party who was going to go for his third knee surgery about the placebo effect, he said, 'Maybe placebos work for psychological things like mild pain, but I can show you my knee X-ray, there is physical mechanical damage. Placebos can't help those.' He may be correct, that the physical damage to his knee is much worse than the physical damage done to Bruce Moseley's patients, but statistically the chances are that his problem was no more severe than Moseley's patients. More importantly, his response implies two beliefs:

- That 'physical' problems with his knee were completely different from 'psychological' things like beliefs.
- That a part of the body is isolated from the whole, much like the part of a machine.

Both of these beliefs have some truth, but are generally mistaken. The mind and body are intimately connected and the body's different parts are connected to each other. Both of these false beliefs can be traced back to the French philosopher and mathematician René Descartes.

Minds, bodies and machines: Descartes' legacy

The idea that placebos can cure 'psychological' things like pain and depression but not 'physiological' ones like damaged knees only makes sense if we separate the psychological – the mind – from the physiological – the body. The idea that the mind and body are separate is quite new and was developed by Descartes. You may have heard this song as a child:

> Row, row, row your boat
> Gently down the stream
> Merrily, merrily, merrily, merrily
> Life is but a dream

As a child, I thought about it and wondered whether we were dreaming that we were alive. I asked my mother whether we were only dreaming, and she said she just knew she was not dreaming. I kept asking *how* she knew and never got a satisfactory answer. Kids are great philosophers, because they always ask why. Descartes used that same trick to investigate what he knew for sure and what he was not sure about – what he might be dreaming about.

After asking himself why a few dozen times, he became convinced that he couldn't even be sure he had a body – he might be dreaming that he had a body. He could, however, be sure that he had a *mind*, because you need a mind to dream and think. That is when he said, 'I think therefore I am'. A consequence of Descartes' inspiration about having a mind but not a body led him to separate the mind and body. The idea that the mind and body were separate was revolutionary at the time, because people at that time believed that minds, souls or 'vital forces' were part of the body. That is why before Descartes' idea took hold, people did not see a contradiction in things such as faith healing and holy water, which allegedly cured many ailments.

Unfortunately for Descartes, his idea that the mind and body are separate does not stand up to common sense. If they could be separated, then:

- How could alcohol, which acts on your body, change your mind?
- How could antidepressant drugs, which are physical things, improve your mood?
- How come being in physical pain can make you depressed?

The mind/body connection provides a basis for accepting how placebo surgery can improve 'physical' symptoms, how relaxing your body can relax your mind (and vice versa) and, as we will see in the upcoming chapters, how positive thoughts can trigger your body to produce endorphins and dopamine that make your body feel good.

To be fair to Descartes, he admitted that the mind and body interacted, but once he had separated them, he had trouble explaining adequately how they could interact. In spite of the fact that common sense tells us that the mind and body are intimately connected, we still continue to speak as though some things are 'just psychological' and others are physical or mechanical (and not psychological). I am not sure why this is the case. I suspect one reason is that most societies have become secular, and science has done away with souls and other invisible things, so the only option is to see bodies as soul-less machines.

Talking about machines, Descartes had another idea that continues to make it difficult for us to see how the mind can influence the body. He thought the body was a machine. If the body is a machine, it is natural to look at one part of the body, such as the knee, in isolation. If part of a machine is faulty, we fix it. There is no point worrying about the machine 'as a whole', let alone how a mind influences it.

Descartes was not entirely wrong to say that we are machines. Our heart is like a pump, our muscles and bones act like pulleys and levers, and even drugs seem to work on cells the way a mini tool might work on a tiny machine. Taking the body to be a machine has led to many advances in surgery and medicine. At a general level, however, your body is more than a machine.

You are more than the sum of your parts

You might try to describe someone by describing how tall they are, what colour their skin and hair is, what their voice sounds like, and how beautiful their eyes, nose, lips and legs are. This would be good, but it misses something about them as a whole person. For example (God forbid), the person you describe gets in an accident and has to have their legs amputated and they get bad burns. Now they will not be as tall, and they will look different. Yet in essence, they would still be the same person. There is something more to us than our parts.

If a part of a machine is broken, you can fix it and it does not affect the other parts too much. Not so with the body. In order to maintain what scientists call 'homeostasis' (basically: balance), different systems need to work together. To survive, the body needs to maintain the right body temperature, breathing rate and heart rate. So when the body temperature falls, blood vessels contract to preserve heat, shivering is induced to make muscles more active (and produce more heat), and you stop sweating. This makes the body temperature rise. If the body temperature gets too high, blood vessels get bigger to release more heat, and you sweat to cool off. All these systems: blood vessels dilating, sweat glands giving off fluid or not, and shivering, are connected, so when you affect one you affect the other. Yet the pictures in scientific magazines often make it appear as though there are isolated systems.

In addition to being connected, the parts of the body are linked in often unknown ways. Take the example of unpredicted drug effects. In 2006, a drug called TGN1412 was first tested on six healthy volunteers, who were paid £2,000 (about $2,500) each to participate in the trial. The first time that drugs are used with humans, scientists use tiny doses for safety reasons. In the first TGN1412 trial, the dose used in the humans was five hundred times lower than that found to be safe and effective in monkeys.

Yet within minutes of being given these very low doses, the white blood cells in the human volunteers disappeared. This led to catastrophic organ failure with the victims fighting for their lives, over a month of hospitalisation, and likely permanent damage to their immune systems that will leave them vulnerable to disease for the rest of their lives. One of the victims lost all his toes and the tips of all his fingers. Not only did the drug operate differently in animals than in humans (which is obvious to many people) but the extremely serious organ failure was not predicted by scientists who had studied how the drug activated various bodily parts for many years.

In addition to activating the system they thought it would activate, the drug also acted on other parts with disastrous consequences. Different parts of the patients' bodies were connected in ways that the scientists didn't predict.

More rarely, drugs can have surprising positive effects. For example, Sildenafil, originally developed to reduce chest pain, did not have much of an effect for this in trials. However, researchers at the drug company Pfizer, who owned it, noticed that many of the middle-aged men in the trial were asking for more because it improved their sex lives dramatically. The drug was subsequently marketed as Viagra and became a huge commercial success. Again, the reason for the surprising effect was that Viagra activated an unsuspected mechanism in men's reproductive organs.

Besides being hopelessly interconnected, two things tie your body *as a whole* together, and make it difficult for the health of an individual part to be viewed in isolation. These two things are *life* and *consciousness*. The fact that your body is alive cannot be explained by looking at the atoms and molecules or any other parts that make up your body. Your body is composed of Oxygen (65 per cent), Carbon (18 per cent), Hydrogen (10 per cent), Nitrogen (3 per cent), Calcium (1.5 per cent), Phosphorus (1 per cent), Potassium (0.5 per cent), and one per cent other stuff such as boron, chromium, cobalt, copper, fluorine, iodine and iron.

You can buy these chemicals for a few dollars at a chemical factory. What is it about the arrangement of these chemicals that makes you alive? What it means to be alive has perplexed scientists and philosophers for centuries, and there is no straightforward answer. Yet we cannot talk about the body or its parts without mentioning life, which ties everything together.

Consciousness also ties our entire bodies together. Live humans, and probably many other animals, are conscious. If you are reading these words and you are aware that you are reading them, then you are conscious. When you taste food, you are conscious. If you get knocked out or you are in a coma you are still alive, but you are not really aware and something central is missing from your life. Consciousness is fundamental to the idea of being alive. Scientists and philosophers have been chasing their tails for centuries trying to discover what and where it is. They have looked everywhere in the body and can't find it. They can find things in our brains that are correlated with our experience (for example, a part of the brain lights up when we see a dog), but they have not explained our experience of seeing a dog.

Not wanting to invoke souls or vital forces, scientists came up with 'emergent properties' to explain life and consciousness. A good example of an emergent property is water. Water is made up of hydrogen and oxygen atoms. At room temperature both oxygen and hydrogen are highly flammable gases. Water is composed of oxygen and hydrogen, but is a liquid at room temperature and is pretty much the opposite of flammable. You cannot predict what water is like no matter how hard you stare at oxygen and hydrogen atoms. The wetness of water *emerges* out of the combination of hydrogen and oxygen atoms.

Consciousness and life can also be described as emergent properties. According to the emergent property point of view, life emerges from the body's organisation of molecules, cells and organs. Scientists and philosophers say that emergence is scientific and not mysterious in the way souls and vital forces are. The emergence story makes sense, but it is unclear how using the word 'emergence' helps explain the nature of life. Leading experts have been trying for decades to define why emergence is more scientific than older concepts like souls and vital forces. It is fair to say that the jury is still out regarding the extent to which they have succeeded.

I don't really care if people call life and consciousness emergent properties or something else. The fact is that there is something about your whole body that makes it alive, which connects all your body's parts together. And – what is more relevant to understanding placebo surgery – where you direct your consciousness (such as towards positive thoughts) can affect your body.

Conclusion: Putting Descartes' legacy into perspective

Understanding that your body is more than just a machine, and that your mind and body are connected, makes it much easier to understand how placebo surgery works. The reason people think that surgery is the best treatment for 'purely mechanical' knee or back problems is that they view the knee or vertebra as isolated parts of the body. The wound-healing cascade shows how the different parts of the body can reorganise themselves to compensate for, and even heal, damage done to the knee or back.

Placebo surgery can also work because we expect it to work: our minds can influence our bodies. And as we will see in the forthcoming chapters, the mind can induce the body to produce its own painkillers and anti-inflammatories. This doesn't mean that thinking positive thoughts will immediately cure all the diseases in the world. It does not mean our cars can run on Earl Grey tea if only we wish it deeply enough. But as Dan Moerman said in the quote at the beginning of this book, 'people are not machines, and we shouldn't treat them as such'.

Takeaway 1: Make sure your decision to have back, hip or knee surgery is evidence based

Unless you are an extreme case, discuss with your doctor the possibility of conservative management before opting for back, hip or knee surgery. Systematic reviews have shown that surgery is rarely better than conservative management for these problems (including many types of fractures). Conservative management means doing physiotherapy and other lifestyle interventions such as exercise and improving diet. Go back to the dialogue at the end of Chapter Two and have an open, two-way conversation with your doctor.

The relaxation exercises from this book and (appropriate) yoga have also been shown to help with back, knee and hip problems. There are two big advantages of conservative therapy over surgery. First, it does not have the side effects of surgery. A quarter of patients undergoing surgery experience side effects including fractures, heart disease, trouble breathing, blood clots, stroke, additional operations, and even death. Second, conservative management is much cheaper, which is better for your pocket. Even if you live in a country with a national health service, you still save money, because it will affect how much tax you pay.

Takeaway 2: Use your mind to control your body, and vice versa

This exercise is easy and fun. To do it, you will have to read through it once and then try it. Whether you are standing up or sitting down, hunch your shoulders forward and look down at the ground. Stay in that position and imagine a scale from one to ten. Ten means 'never felt better' and one means 'never felt worse'. What number would you give yourself on that scale? Remember that number. Now sit up tall with your shoulders back and chest sticking out. Even if you have to fake it, put a little smile on your face. Thinking of the same scale, where one means you feel terrible and ten means you never felt better – now where do you rank yourself?

Remember the number. Is it higher than the number you gave yourself when you hunched over? By far the vast majority of people find that they feel quite a bit better. Even feeling a few points higher means that simple exercise had the same effect as some drugs. So the next time you need a little boost, just stand or sit up straight, and smile (even if you have to fake it). Now think . . . could a machine do that and feel the same way?

Takeaway 3: Avoid the blame game

Here is a mistaken line of reasoning that I sometimes hear:

- If thoughts can make you feel better, then you just need to choose positive thoughts and you will not be sick.
- And since you are in control of your thoughts, it is your fault if you are sick.

This line of reasoning is wrong. It is true that thoughts can influence your health; however, so does your body. I was born with jaundice and that had nothing to do with my thoughts. Simply because the body and mind are connected, it does not mean that the mind controls everything about the body. The body is a key player on the team, too. So it is wrong to say that if you are sick, it is only because you are thinking the wrong thoughts.

Also, just because thinking positive thoughts will make us feel better, it doesn't mean that doing so is easy. In the same way that people's bodies are different, so are their thought patterns. Some people, like Khamis Elessi and Alice Herz-Sommers (mentioned in Chapter Six), are naturally more optimistic than others. I would say I have average optimism and sometimes I find it difficult to be positive but my negative thoughts rarely lead to depression or failure to get on with life. Other people I know are negative no matter what. For whatever reason – genetics, upbringing, and other experiences – we have developed our own thought patterns and it is as hard to change these as making our biceps bigger. It is easiest to understand the difficulty in altering our thought patterns if we acknowledge the reality and importance of the mind.

There is a bigger reason why it makes no sense to believe that your health is your fault. When you blame someone, you are not making them happy. As we are all connected to other people (more about this in Part IV of this book), making someone else unhappy will have an adverse effect on us.

Since you are someone, you also should not blame yourself if you might find it difficult to modify your thoughts and habits. Avoid the blame game.

PART III

A Closer Look at Your Inner Healer

I said that the cure itself is a certain leaf, but in addition to the drug there is a certain charm, which if someone chants when he makes use of it, the medicine altogether restores him to health, but without the charm there is no profit from the leaf.

Plato

To the pharmaceutical industry, placebos are annoying hurdles that they have to jump over to prove their drugs work. To sceptics, placebos are fake medicine that tricksters exploit to sell phony cures. Meanwhile, debate rages about whether placebos actually work. Some think they are powerful cures for almost everything, while others say they are useless. Amid these debates, one thing is certain: most doctors use them. Surveys of doctors in the US, Germany and Israel show that over half of doctors admit to having prescribed them at least once. In the UK, as I mentioned in the Introduction, my 2013 survey showed that ninety-seven per cent of doctors have prescribed placebos at least once.

Maybe these doctors know instinctively what my systematic review of placebo effects showed: placebos can be powerful. Sometimes doctors use sugar pills or salt water injections as placebos. In one case, I heard a story from a doctor who told me about a known drug addict who came into his office complaining of back pain. The patient begged for morphine to kill the pain; however, my colleague knew that additional morphine was not good for the patient, so he gave him a salt water injection but pretended it was morphine. It seemed to work.

More frequently, doctors use things like antibiotics for viral diseases (so the antibiotics have no effect), or low doses of medications that are so low they have no pharmacological effect. Using an antibiotic for a known viral infection, or a tiny dose of a treatment that has no pharmacological effect, is in many ways no different from a placebo.

In the next few chapters we will see that researchers have

revealed a great deal about how they work. Taking a placebo gives the patient some reason to believe they will feel better soon. The belief in a positive outcome helps the body produce its own feel-good chemicals. Positive beliefs also help to reduce anxiety, pain and depression. Our brains can learn to associate certain environments like doctors' offices and hospitals with good outcomes. These associations that our brain make help to explain how 'open-label' placebos – placebos patients know are placebos – work. A doctor's attention and friendly manner can also have a positive health effect on their patient. All of these things can interact to take the brake off the immune system.

8

The Power of Positive Thinking

*Whether you think you can, or whether you think you can't,
you're right*

Henry Ford

Professor George Lewith is a family doctor who shares my interest in placebo research. He is also one of the nicest and most helpful people I know. Soon after we first met at a conference, I decided to ask him for some advice about a back problem that started when I was a rower. It was not an emergency, so there was no need for me to go to the hospital, but it was Saturday afternoon and I did not want to disturb George on the weekend. I didn't think he would take the call, so I called his mobile number with the intention of leaving him a message. I was surprised when he answered.

'Great to hear from you, Jeremy,' he said. 'How are you?'

'Very well, thanks, how are you?'

'I'm really happy, because I'm at the hospital where my grandson has just been born,' he answered.

Shit, I thought, not only did I call him at the weekend, but I interrupted his special family time. I took a deep breath and said, 'Let me call you back, because my question is not very important.' But he insisted that he had time to talk, listened to my question, and gave me a helpful answer. I thanked him, thinking what a nice guy he was.

'It's my pleasure,' he said. Then he added, 'Feel free to call me any time you have a question.' And he meant it, because I have called him since whenever I have a medical question and he always takes the time to answer.

133

George's colleagues know that he is very nice to his patients, too. But some of them think that spending so much time and energy being pleasant and positive is a waste, and that he should focus on prescribing the right drugs.

One of his colleagues, a doctor called Bruce Thomas, told George that his kindness might give patients a warm, fuzzy feeling, but it did not make them get better. Dr Thomas knew all about pathology and physiology, but he clearly did not believe that the doctor's bedside manner was all that important. In 1987, George challenged Bruce to try being positive with his patients to see what happened. Dr Thomas accepted the challenge, presumably thinking he would prove George was wrong.

For his trial, Dr Thomas prepared a series of cards and wrote *positive* on half of them and *negative* on the other half. Then he shuffled the cards and put them in a drawer in his desk. As patients came to visit him, he first diagnosed them to see whether he believed they had a life-threatening ailment that needed referral to a specialist or an ambulance. If not, he reached into his drawer to draw a card.

- **Positive consultation.** If the card indicated he should provide a positive consultation, Dr Thomas gave the patient a firm diagnosis and confidently told him or her they would be better within a few days. If no prescription was given, the patient was informed that it was because none was required. If a prescription was given, Dr Thomas told the patient confidently that the treatment would surely make them better soon.
- **Negative consultation.** If Dr Thomas chose a *negative* card, he would tell the patients, 'I cannot be certain what is the matter with you.' If no treatment was prescribed, the following words were added, 'And therefore I will give you no treatment.' If a treatment was prescribed, the patient was told, 'I am not sure that the treatment I am going to give you will have an effect.'

134

Dr Thomas did this until he had treated one hundred patients with negative consultations and one hundred patients with positive consultations. He found that sixty-four per cent of the patients who received positive consultations got better within two weeks, whereas only thirty-nine per cent of the patients with negative consultations got better. That means patients who left their consultation with firm, confident diagnoses were about twice as likely to get better than those who Dr Thomas had left with less confidence about their prospects. Dr Thomas called the resulting research paper, 'Is there a point in being positive?'

One problem with Dr Thomas's study was that the outcomes were subjective, because it was up to the patients to report whether they got better or not. It is possible that some of the patients might have *said* they got better, when in fact they did not feel any better. After Dr Thomas told them with so much certainty that they would feel better, they might have felt scared of contradicting him. Yet dozens of studies conducted since then with more robust and objective outcomes have confirmed that there is a point in being positive.

Fabrizio Benedetti, a famous placebo researcher based in Italy, compared what he called *open* and *hidden* treatments. Patients treated *openly* knew they were getting a treatment and so expected to get better. Patients in the *hidden* group did not know they were being treated and so did not expect to get better. Normally you cannot give a treatment to a patient without them knowing, but Benedetti thought of a clever way to get around that problem.

In the hospital where he works, a lot of thoracotomy operations are performed. A thoracotomy involves cutting through the chest wall to access the heart and lungs. They are usually performed to remove tumours, confirm diagnosis of a lung or chest disease, re-inflate collapsed tissue, or remove fluid from the chest. Forty-two such patients were already connected intravenously to fluid bags at the hospital.

All the patients in Benedetti's study received morphine

through the pre-connected intravenous line, but only half of them were told that they were being given it. Doctors informed these patients they were receiving a powerful painkiller, before telling them their pain would go away within a few minutes. The remaining twenty-one patients were not told they were receiving the same morphine dose, and use of programmable intravenous devices meant no doctor or nurses entered their room.

Patients in both groups were asked to rate their pain in a diary thirty minutes and sixty minutes after receiving the morphine, using a ten-point scale on which zero meant no pain and ten meant unbearable pain. The morphine delivered by a doctor who told patients they were receiving a powerful painkiller was twenty per cent more effective at reducing pain than the hidden administration of morphine.

Benedetti's clever study shows that positive messages from doctors do more than make patients feel better in a subjective, fluffy way. They work to make the patient actually *get* better. Using the same open-versus-hidden treatment design, Benedetti and his colleagues hooked ten patients with Parkinson's disease up to electrodes. They then underwent a procedure called Deep Brain Stimulation (DBS), which is used to help counter the neurological symptoms of the condition. It involves electrical impulses being sent to parts of the brain that control movement to block abnormal nerve signals.

Half of the study participants were told when the electrodes were turned on and half were not. For some reason, researchers often like to use complicated words for simple things. The slowing down of movements in people with Parkinson's is called *bradykinesia*. Before and after their treatment, those in the study underwent a test commonly used to assess bradykinesia in Parkinson's patients. They were asked to move their index fingers to a target in response to a light being switched on. The patients with the *open* stimulation – those told they were receiving DBS – improved their reaction times by twice as much as the patients who received hidden treatment.

In 2017, I conducted a systematic review of sixteen randomised trials on the effects of positive expectations on treatment for pain. These involved almost 4,000 patients, all of whom went through tests similar to the one Dr Thomas did to challenge George's belief.

I concluded that positive messages reduce pain by as much or more than most common drugs for treating pain, but without the side effects. The doctors' positive messages also reduced nausea, asthma symptoms, anxiety and depression. The other thing I found is that positive messages didn't just affect 'soft', 'psychological' outcomes but could affect physical things too. Besides hand movement of Parkinson's patients, trials have showed that lung activity of asthma patients, and how much blood flows through chest pain patients' arteries. The positive messages also reduced the amount of medication patients used and reduced their length of stay in hospital. But how do positive expectations work?

The benefits of chilling out

Positive messages can lead to health benefits in many ways. The first is through the reduction of stress and anxiety. If you think something really bad is going to happen, like your cold might be serious pneumonia, your headache might be a tumour, or your back pain will paralyse you, you are likely to become anxious. As we saw earlier, anxiety and stress increase the risk of suffering heart disease and many other conditions. Several trials also show that depression is more likely and pain levels higher in those suffering from anxiety. This seems to be because anxiety causes the release of a hormone called cholecytoskinin, which increases the intensity of pain messages from the body to the brain. If a doctor reassures you that everything is going to be okay (which it usually is), or that they have a plan (in case it really is something that needs to be dealt with more seriously), your anxiety is likely to be reduced, and this can reduce your pain.

Expectations and dopamine

Imagine you are a caveman just back from your very first buffalo hunt. You noticed that the caveman whose spear hit the buffalo got a 'high five' (or whatever the caveman equivalent was). You like the idea of getting a caveman high five, but the next hunt is more difficult. You get close to your target, but the herd hears you and stampedes away. You have to circle a long way around to approach them from downwind. After a day of walking with barely any food or water, you are tired. Your head sags, your feet are bleeding, and your body is telling you to lie down and sleep. The only thing that keeps you going is the group of older, more experienced hunters, who keep pushing you forward. After what seems like many hours of walking, you look up to see the buffalo within striking distance. Remembering your desire for the caveman high five, you get a surge of energy. You forget you are tired, sneak quietly up to the fearsome animals and launch your spear. Hit in the neck, a buffalo tries to run, but stumbles, falls and dies. Triumphant, you accept your hard-won caveman high five, and experience another energy boost.

The energy boosts you just received came from the brain's reward system, which basically makes us feel good when we do things that help us survive. Things like getting food, earning money, or engaging in activities that help you produce healthy offspring are good for your survival. One way the brain rewards you is by increasing the amount of dopamine in your body. Dopamine feels good, and makes you want to do more stuff that increases your survival prospects. You can also get that good feeling by thinking about something good happening. That is one reason why the caveman got a rush when he got near the buffalo and thought about actually killing it.

If dopamine sounds like the kind of thing you can get addicted to, that's because it is. It is the reason we can become addicted to things like food, sex and money. While these things are good for our survival *up to a point*, they are detrimental beyond that point. And if we are honest, most of us indulge in at least one of these a bit too much. We often eat past the point we are full, work past the point where we have earned enough money, and keep lusting beyond the point where we have had enough. Many illegal recreational drugs target the reward system. Cocaine, for example, boosts dopamine levels in your body by preventing the brain from reabsorbing it.

Dopamine also explains why a positive expectation reduced Parkinson's symptoms in Benedetti's study. One cause of Parkinson's disease is when the part of the brain that produces dopamine stops working properly. In one study, patients with the condition were given either apomorphine, which increases dopamine levels, or placebo, but were not told which group they were in. The results were striking: dopamine activity in both groups increased two hundred per cent. The patients given the placebo thought they were getting the real drug, which caused them to expect a positive reward and increased the amount of dopamine in their bodies. Drugs for Parkinson's often work in precisely the same way.

Pharmaceutical therapies for some other conditions also work by increasing dopamine levels. For example, psychostimulants are used to treat ADHD increase dopamine and norepinephrine levels in the brain.

Dopamine is not the only drug your body produces when you think positive thoughts or when doctors tell you to expect success.

Expectations and endorphins

The expectation of a positive reward also produces endorphins, which are a natural form of the painkilling drug morphine. In another one of his cool studies, Fabrizio Benedetti gave people placebo treatments that he said were powerful treatments, giving them a positive expectation. Along with the placebo treatments, he gave some of them a drug called naloxone. Naloxone stops morphine and endorphins working. He then used a tourniquet to cause all the study participants some pain. The people to whom he gave placebos experienced less pain that those who got the placebos plus naloxone. Benedetti's study showed that the naloxone had blocked the effects of positive expectations. This proved that positive expectations cause the body to produce endorphins.

Positive expectations make you change your behaviour

At high school, I was one of those kids who got good grades but got picked last when we were playing team sports. When I went on to study engineering at Dartmouth College in New Hampshire, I admired my popular athletic peers, but saw myself as a geek. Thankfully, one day I bumped into the university's new rowing coach (I literally bumped into him), who was out on campus approaching any students six foot or taller to ask if they would try out for the team. I was just over six feet tall so he told me and his other potential new recruits that we were going to be really fast rowers. As fast as we wanted, in fact.

Being tall is a big advantage in rowing and at just over six feet tall, I am on the short side for the sport. So I was not that great a candidate to be very good at it. But I didn't know any better, and I also admired and trusted the coach, so I trained hard. Very hard. I often did two sessions per day each one lasting between one and two hours. Had I not believed I was going to be good, I would not have endured the gut-wrenching agony of those sessions. Thanks to the hard training, I became a pretty good rower. Academics, who love impressive-sounding jargon, call believing that you can achieve your goals *self-efficacy*. I prefer the term self-belief. Having a positive self-belief motivates you to do things (in my case, train hard).

Belief in our ability to achieve our goals can have other effects, beyond improving rowing ability. As I said earlier, research shows back pain can be lessened through exercise. Sometimes this can feel like tough love: painful but good for you. And motivating ourselves to do exercise even if we do not have back pain is challenging. If you have negative expectations and say to yourself, 'It is never going to get better,' you might not bother doing any exercise at all, which usually makes the pain worse. The same goes for quitting smoking: if you think it is impossible, why try to begin with? You need to believe you can to even try!

Since diet and exercise can reduce the risk of diseases like diabetes, heart disease, cancer and obesity, the belief that you can improve what you eat and do more exercise can actually lower the risk of developing these conditions. Take diabetes: research has shown that it can be prevented and its symptoms can be lessened through exercise. Of course, it is a lot easier to plan to go jogging more often, eat more lettuce and cut out chocolate bars, than it is to do these beneficial things. But if you expect to get better as a result, you are more likely to be able to motivate yourself to achieve your goals. And when you stick to the healthy programme, your diabetic symptoms will be reduced.

Self-belief is important, because it is not always easy to change our behaviour, even when we know it is good for us. I find it difficult to motivate myself to eat fewer sweet things. Ever since I was a small child, I have liked sugary snacks and even now my co-workers know they should keep the cookies out of my sight or they disappear. Once I almost convinced myself that I had a gene that made me have a special desire to eat chocolate cake and other sweet things. However genes *determine* those things – more about that in Chapter Thirteen. The fact is that my belief I could stop eating sugar actually helped me stop. Besides positive beliefs, it often helps to have friends who tell you that you can achieve things you find difficult.

How someone else's belief in us can help

The Pygmalion experiment discussed in Chapter Two demonstrated how teachers' beliefs about students can affect these students' performance. At least seventeen trials have replicated the original Pygmalion experiment in teaching, leadership and management.

Pygmalion effects also occur in medicine. In one of a number of trials that have shown this, sixty-three elderly residents at six nursing homes were given a comprehensive check of their mental health and of their physical abilities. They were then randomly assigned to a 'high-expectancy' or 'average-expectancy' condition. Nurses were told that the elderly people in the high-expectancy group would recover more quickly and respond better to treatment.

After three months, a researcher, who did not know to which group the participants had been assigned, gave them another check-up. Those in the high-expectancy group did better in three out of the four outcomes measured: they were less depressed, were less likely to be admitted to the hospital, and had higher mental status than the average-expectancy group. They only did worse in one of the outcomes: the high-expectancy group needed more assistance from nurses than the other patients.

The way Pygmalion effects work in medicine is probably similar to how they work in a school. If a doctor believes they are prescribing a treatment that is really going to help a patient, they might treat him or her differently to someone else being given a placebo. Because of their belief that the patient is going to get better, they might be more encouraging, which could give the patient positive expectations. On the other hand, if the doctor believes that a patient is being given a 'mere' placebo, they might communicate less confidence about the outcome and generate negative expectations.

How negative expectations harm: nocebo effects

In the same way that positive expectations can lead to positive outcomes, negative expectations can lead to negative outcomes. This has been demonstrated in research on the pain children experience when doctors give them injections. In one such study, doctors were asked to tell their young patients either 'This is going to hurt' or 'This might hurt a bit'. A third group of doctors gave children their injections while their mothers distracted them.

The children were much more likely to cry when the doctor said that the needle would hurt because they *expected* the pain. When the mother was distracting the child, the child had no expectations and did not feel as much pain. This shows how doctors who use negative words can exacerbate symptoms.

A group of researchers in China compared the effect of no words to negative words in more than five hundred patients who had hysterectomies (a surgical procedure to remove the womb or part of it). The patients all had a syringe containing painkilling drugs attached to their intravenous lines. They had access to a Patient Controlled Analgesia (PCA) pump that allowed them to increase the amount of painkiller they received when they felt more pain. Half of the patients received negative messages from the doctors such as, 'Please, it was useless, do not trust the PCA pump.' The other half of the patients were not subjected to negative messages.

The researchers then measured how much pain participants experienced, as well as how much morphine they asked for. The group who received the negative messages – and hence had negative expectations – reported feeling more pain and required more morphine than the control patients. Those patients who were not told that using the PCA pump was bad took an average of 45 milligrams of morphine over two days, whereas the negative-messages group consumed an average of 72 milligrams – an increase of more than sixty per cent. An average difference of 27 milligrams of morphine is a lot, given that the suggested dose of morphine for adults is 5 to 20 milligrams.

Several systematic reviews have confirmed that negative expectations can harm. Colleagues of mine at Oxford University have started to investigate in more detail how negative expectations work. It seems that the expectation of a negative outcome activates brain regions associated with feeling pain.

Negative words also increase patients' anxiety and stress levels, which can have negative health impacts. While placebos have beneficial effects because of positive beliefs, the *nocebo effect* is the scientific term for the harms caused by negative words, and is the result of negative expectations and beliefs.

A problem is that most of us have too many negative thoughts. Even people who think of themselves as optimistic are more pessimistic than they think. One cool study asked people the following questions:

- Who will have a heart attack first: you or your colleagues?
- Who will retire with more money: you or your peers?
- Who is more likely to get into drugs: your kids or your neighbours' kids?

Most people said their colleagues would have a heart attack before them, that they would retire with more money than their peers, and that their neighbours' kids would be more likely to take drugs than their own. But this can't be right, because on average half of us will end up better and half worse than our peers. Although we appear to be more positive than we have the right to be, we also have a lot of negative thoughts. It is hard to capture thoughts in a way that can be measured, but when scientists try to do this, they find many to be negative.

Dr Raj Raghunathan reports studies showing that two out of three of our spontaneous thoughts are negative. Dr

Raghunathan did a bit more digging into the kinds of negative thoughts people had and found that they fall into three main categories:

1. Thoughts related to inferiority ('Other students are going to do better than me in the exam.')
2. Thoughts related to love and approval ('How come I am the only one who's not taken?')
3. Thoughts related to control seeking ('Why don't my teammates ever listen to the suggestions I make?').

I am sure we all catch ourselves having these types of negative thoughts from time to time. Some negative people say they are only being realistic and honest about life, and to them life is bad, so they're just telling the 'truth'. It is true that the world can be terrible sometimes. However, just like the teachers' expectations in the Pygmalion experiment made students perform *better*, having negative thoughts and expectations can make things worse than they would otherwise have been.

The good thing about these negative thoughts is that they can be changed. Thoughts of inferiority come from society telling us it is important to excel (which literally means to rise above others). This leads to constant comparison and inferiority feelings, because there is always someone bigger and better (and also worse!). Negative thoughts about love arise from the fact we are told that life without a 'soul mate' is not worthwhile, which is not so. And thoughts about control come from the false idea that you can control the world. Since the sources of many of these negative thoughts come from learned beliefs, it means that we can, with some effort, unlearn them. Before suggesting how, I am going to show you how medical bureaucrats who see themselves as guardians of patient safety force negative beliefs down patients' throats.

How the wrong type of informed consent can cause harm

Have you ever read about the possible side effects of aspirin? According to the NHS, common ones include:

- indigestion
- stomach aches
- bleeding or bruising more easily than normal

The rare side effects include:

- hives (an itchy rash)
- tinnitus (hearing sounds that come from inside your body)
- asthma attacks
- allergic reaction that causes breathing problems, swelling of the mouth, and a sudden rash
- stomach bleeding, including vomiting blood
- bleeding in the brain

Scary, right? That is why we don't read the small print. While we probably take too much aspirin, millions of people take aspirin without their brains bleeding. Reading about the multiple and varied side effects can induce stress. While it is important for some people to know about these, most of us can take aspirin safely without worrying.

People who enrol in clinical trials are forced to read the small print. Doctors and researchers involved in trials must inform patients about all the potential benefits *and* side effects of a new treatment, no matter how small the risks involved, in order for participants to be able to give their full, informed consent. A review of trials of Parkinson's disease and depression treatments showed that between five per cent and ten per cent of the patients who took the placebo treatment dropped out of the trials, usually due to side effects. But the placebo treatment could not possibly have caused the side effects. They can only have been caused by negative beliefs.

Unfortunately, current ethical regulations require patients to be fully informed, even if the patients do not want to know all the gory details. This is crazy and needs to change. My colleague and friend Sir Iain Chalmers proposed a model for informed consent that is interactive and responds to the needs and wishes of patients. It would go something like this:

Good morning, Mrs Jones, my name is Dr Smith. Please sit down and make yourself comfortable. Your general practitioner has probably explained to you that he has asked me to see you because your breathlessness doesn't seem to be getting any better, and he wondered whether I might be able to suggest ways of helping. I hope I will be able to do so, but this may well mean seeing you on several occasions over the next few months and working together to find the best treatment for your condition.

I'm more likely to be able to help if I can get to know more about you and your priorities and preferences. As this is the first time we've met, I thought it might be helpful to mention briefly how I will try to do this. Patients vary in the amount of information that they want to give and receive from their doctors. Most patients seem to get less information from their doctors than they want, but others would rather not be told some of the things that some doctors assume that they must want to know. Because you and I don't know each other yet, I'm going to need your help in learning how much information you want about your problem, and about the possible treatment options.

I'm going to depend on you to prompt me to give you more information if you think I'm not being sufficiently forthcoming, or to tell me that you've heard enough if you think I'm overdoing it. You also need to know that I will never lie in response to a straight question from you, and if I don't know the answer I will do my best to find it for you. Does that seem to you to be an acceptable way of proceeding?

One randomised trial has found this model of informed consent reduces the side effects patients suffer compared to when they are forced to worry about unusual and rare side effects. These studies show that negative words have negative health effects.

Takeaway (for doctors and healthcare practitioners): Positive words for your patients

Here is a sample of words that were used by clinicians in randomised trials that were shown to have a positive effect on patients, especially for pain.

- 'You will be better within a week or so.'
- 'An active medication that has been shown to be effective for some types of pain will be tested.'
- 'The agent you have just been given is known to power-fully reduce pain in some patients.'
- 'The PCA pump was very effective in removing the post-operative pain affliction.'

Takeaway (for everyone): Three things you can do to replace negative thoughts with positive ones

You can be your own doctor and give yourself the same messages as above – some studies show that reading positive messages (even if a doctor does not give them to you) can reduce pain. Modify the words for doctors listed above so that you are talking about yourself. For example:

- 'I will be better within a week or so.'
- 'I will feel better within four weeks.'
- 'This will work for me.'

Dealing with negative thoughts (such as the opposite of the statements above) is also important . . . but challenging. If I knew an easy way to banish all negative thoughts from me

– or you – I would tell you. So I will just share three tools that have helped me. The second one is based on positive psychology exercises, which, as I mentioned earlier, is supported by systematic review evidence.

1. **Throw them away**. Write the negative thought down on a piece of paper, crumple it up, and slam-dunk the paper into the garbage. Imagine those negative thoughts flowing away with it.

2. **The letter of compassion exercise**. Write yourself a letter of self-compassion in which you show understanding and are nice to yourself. Remember you are only human. Choose an aspect of yourself that you dislike or are prone to criticise. It could be appearance, career or relationships – anything. Now:

   • Write in detail about how that makes you feel. Describe the thoughts, images, emotions and stories that come up when you think of this.

   • Now imagine someone real or imaginary who loves you unconditionally, who is completely supportive and accepting. This person only sees potential in you, they see anything you perceive as 'negative' as an opportunity to grow. They love you for who you are, and they embrace you kindly.

   • Now write a letter from this kind person to you. What does he or she say? How do they encourage you to grow? Write freely without worrying about the grammar and structure of the letter.

After you complete the letter, put it aside for a few minutes. Then read it. Let the words sink in. Feel the encouragement, support, compassion and acceptance. Read the letter whenever you feel down about that aspect of your life. Remember: accepting yourself is the first step towards making a positive change.

3. **Fuck it**. If all else fails, fuck it. A couple called John Parkin and Gaia Pollini tried all meditation and other techniques for decades and still could not get rid of their negative thoughts. Nothing worked for them. In the end they were so exhausted by trying to do all the things gurus were advising them to do that they said 'fuck it'. Just saying that made them feel relaxed and positive. Now they even offer 'Fuck it therapy'. Twitter users who do not fancy splashing out on one of the Fuck It retreats that Parkin and Pollini run in Italy can get daily doses of fuck it philosophy by following @thefuckitlife. Next time you feel frustrated because things are not going your way, or because of a thought you don't like, say 'fuck it'. Think of it as a naughty mantra.

9

Conditioning: Awakening the Body's Inner Pharmacy

The decision to believe or not believe is not entirely in our hands. I might be happier and have better manners if I thought I were descended from the emperors of China, but no effort of will on my part can make me believe it, any more than I can will my heart to stop beating.

Steven Weinberg, American physicist
and Nobel laureate

Our subconscious beliefs

People who know me now think of me as a good athlete but, as I mentioned earlier, when I was in high school nobody wanted me in his or her team. I was clumsy and did not really believe I could be a winner at any sport. I remember one day when I was fifteen years old, playing basketball one Saturday morning at the YMCA in my home town of Westmount in Quebec, Canada. Usually in basketball a player in one team will follow a player on the other team to try and prevent them from scoring or getting a pass. I was playing so badly that the guy on the other team, who was supposed to be following me, left me alone to do what I wanted. Instead he would normally cover Justin, the best player in my team, who used to pick me for his team because he was a nice guy.

So on the odd occasion when I had the ball, nobody in the opposing team would try to stop me, allowing me an open shot on the net. Despite being unmarked, I would be so nervous that I frequently missed. I don't know why I was so clumsy and nervous, but I think it was partly down to my first gym teacher in high school.

When I first went to high school, I decided to try out for the basketball team. For one thing I was pretty tall and all the cool kids played basketball. It was also a good way to avoid being bullied, as a lot of those in the basketball team bullied the kids who were not. As part of the try-out, the coach asked me to do a lay up, which involves taking a couple of steps, jumping and then hopefully scoring a basket off the backboard. I was so nervous I tried too hard and missed the net. I was not even close.

'You missed,' he said.

'Can I try again?'

'No,' he said.

'Just one more chance.'

'I can't teach you to play ball. You're too goofy.'

The kids waiting for their turn to try out laughed. I walked away and did not try out again. This experience at the hands of an authority figure helped formulate my belief that I was no good at sports.

The rowing coaches I had later on were the opposite of that basketball coach. I had three in a row, Scott Armstrong, Larry Gluckman and Dusan Kovacevic, who really believed in me. They helped me get pretty good at rowing. After a few years of successful rowing, I went back to play basketball at the same Westmount YMCA against the same guys who used to not want to pick me for the team.

Now I hadn't played basketball for a long time, and these guys had been playing several days per week for years. True that I was in better shape than before because of the rowing. But pulling on oars involves little hand-eye coordination and requires you to develop endurance muscles rather than the explosive muscles you need for basketball. So I should have been relatively *worse*. In fact, I was one of the best players in the team that day. How can we explain this? I did not do a randomised trial, so I can only tell you how I felt. Whereas before I was conditioned to feel overly anxious and stressed and like a loser in sports, now I approached any physical activity competition feeling confident. Scott and my other coaches had helped *condition* me to feel confident.

Conditioning can also have medical effects. The best evidence for this comes from trials of open-label placebos.

Open-label placebos

I have mentioned a few times that placebos can work even if patients know they are placebos. This seems mysterious because placebos are thought of as the power of belief. So if we do not believe they are (or might be) real, how could they work? We can now finally solve that mystery.

In the first of the studies that I know of open-label placebos (placebos that patients know are placebos), two Baltimore doctors by the names of Lee Park and Uno Covi gave open-label placebos to fifteen neurotic patients. They presented the placebo pills to the patients and said, 'Many people with your kind of condition have been helped by what are sometimes called sugar pills and we feel that a so-called sugar pill may help you, too'. The patients took the placebos, and many of them got 'quite a bit better' after having the placebo, even though they knew it was a placebo. But since these patients knew the pills were placebos, they could not expect to get better. And if they didn't expect to get better, how did they get better?

The answer is partly that they *did* expect to get better for two reasons. First, the doctors gave them a positive message along with the placebo. The other reason is that the patients did not believe the doctors. After the placebo made them better, they thought the doctors lied and actually gave them the real drug. The Park and Covi study was small, however, and did not have a control group.

More recent, higher-quality studies confirm that open-label placebos can work. As I mentioned in Chapter Four, Ted Kaptchuk of Harvard Medical School randomised eighty patients with severe IBS to receive either no treatment or open-label sugar pill placebos. After a few weeks, Kaptchuk's team compared their scores from the commonly used IBS Global Improvement Scale questionnaire both before and after taking the placebos with those in the no-treatment group. Those in the open-label placebo group improved by fifteen per cent more than those in the control group.

I did a systematic review and found five trials (260 participants) of open label placebos. The trials investigated open-label placebo effects for irritable bowel syndrome (IBS), depression, allergic rhinitis, back pain, and attention deficit hyperactivity disorder (ADHD). The effects were positive for all the trials, and had similar effects to the open-label placebo in Kaptchuk's trial. A problem with these studies is that it is hard to blind the patients. Patients are randomised to either an open-label placebo or no treatment, and they know which group they are in. Yet the consistency of the results in these studies suggests a real effect.

How open-label placebos work

There are two main ways that open-label placebos work. First, they are often given together with a positive suggestion. The doctor tells the patient the pill is just a placebo, but adds that it 'produces significant improvement for patients like you'. This suggestion creates a positive expectation, which can activate the reward mechanisms in the brain and help the body to produce its own painkilling endorphins. But conditioning probably also plays a role in explaining how open-label placebos work. Let me say a word about conditioning.

What do the human immune system and Pavlov's dogs have in common?

Russian psychologist Ivan Pavlov made conditioning theory famous in the late 1800s. Pavlov would ring a bell, then feed his dogs. After repeating the process several times, he changed his procedure. Instead of ringing then feeding, he would simply ring the bell. By that time, of course, the dogs had been conditioned to associate the sound of the bell with eating. So they would start to salivate at the mere sound of the bell, even if there was no food. Hundreds of other studies with animals, humans and even cells have been conducted that support his conditioning theory. Conditioning is most likely the mechanism by which our prehistoric ancestors and even the very first single-celled living beings on the planet learned things.

Something many people do not know is that the human immune system can be conditioned, too. This was first discovered in 1895 by an American researcher called John Noland MacKenzie. He had a thirty-two-year-old female patient who complained of severe asthmatic symptoms during the summer months, especially when she was near flowers. Roses seemed to cause the most severe attacks and her symptoms included red itchy eyes, blocked nose, sneezing, and even fever. Apart from the summer after her only child was born, she was confined to bed for most of August.

She had tried many remedies and even some 'quack' cures without success. Cocaine, which at that time was widely used as medicine as well as recreationally, provided relief for about thirty minutes. Some years ago, a doctor had performed a cautery operation, which involved burning the inside of her nose with a red-hot metal rod. This was enormously painful, but seemed to work for several weeks. When she later asked MacKenzie for another cautery operation, he reminded her how painful the first one had been. She replied that the relief was well worth it.

Dr MacKenzie did the cautery operation. Yet for some reason he did not believe that her fits were really caused by rose pollen. He decided to play a trick on her. He had a fake rose made and hid it behind a screen in his office. When she returned a few weeks after the operation, she reported feeling very well. She told him that earlier that day she had attempted to wear some roses, but she had suffered a reaction and so got rid of them. MacKenzie removed the slight scab from the cautery operation, which was loose in her nostril, and examined her carefully. She had no symptoms or signs of allergies: her throat and nose were completely clear.

Once he established that she had been cured, he produced the fake rose from its hiding place. When she saw it, she sneezed, itched her nose and eyes, and spoke with a hoarse voice. She also reported having trouble breathing and when he examined her throat he found it to be red. Her right nostril was completely blocked. He then told her that the rose was fake and she did not believe it until she examined the counterfeit rose herself. She saw it was a fake, but was happy to learn that the cause of her reaction was 'psychological'. She came to visit him a few days later and buried her nostrils in a large, fragrant bunch of real roses without experiencing any symptoms at all. Her reaction to the fake rose was a conditioned response. Her body learned to react when she saw (what she thought was) a rose.

But how can conditioning have this effect? Allergies are autoimmune diseases, which means they are inappropriate immune-system responses. Runny noses and watering eyes are great for flushing away harmful bacteria and viruses. Inflammation, which causes the nose and throat to get congested, occurs because the immune system is dilating the vessels to let more cells that defend the body access the site of injury. But sometimes the immune system gets things wrong and unnecessarily launches our defences against things such as pollen, despite them being harmless. Dr MacKenzie's patient had somehow been conditioned to launch an immune-system reaction to roses and other flowers, just as Pavlov's dogs were conditioned to salivate upon hearing a bell. Dr MacKenzie's story was revolutionary, because it showed that the immune system can be conditioned.

Later animal studies replicated Dr MacKenzie's findings. In a 1975 rat study, American researchers Robert Ader and

Nicholas Cohen divided rats into different groups. Some groups received a flavoured drink containing saccharin and a drug that suppressed the immune system called cyclophosphamide. After being given this cocktail for several days, Ader and Cohen took out the cyclophosphamide and just gave the rats saccharin-laced water. They found that the saccharin water suppressed the immune system in the rats as if they had swallowed cyclophosphamide along with the saccharin water. This is because the rats' immune systems had become conditioned to be suppressed in response to the taste of saccharin. These studies have been replicated with other animals.

Research has shown that the human immune system can be conditioned, too. In 2002, Dr Marion Goebel and colleagues in Germany gave a group of thirty-four healthy male volunteers capsules containing cyclosporin A every twelve hours for three days. Cyclosporin A is a drug used to suppress the immune systems of patients given an organ transplant. When someone gets an organ from a donor, the body thinks it is a foreign invader and instructs the immune system to attack the donor organ. So doctors give drugs to the person who is receiving the organ, in order to suppress the immune system until the body realises the new organ is okay and is good for them.

Goebel mixed cyclosporin A into a cocktail containing strawberry-and-lavender-flavoured milk. They deliberately chose a weird drink that their participants would not have encountered before. The idea was to teach the men's bodies to connect the strange flavour with immune suppression. In the second phase of the trial, the men continued taking their unusual drink, but this time it contained no cyclosporin A. Throughout the study, Dr Goebel's team measured levels of immune system cells like interleukin-2 and white blood cells. They found the participants' immune systems continued to be suppressed, even once the cyclosporin A had been removed from their flavoured milk.

A few years later, Luana Colloca in Italy showed that sensations of pain can also be conditioned. The forty-six healthy volunteers in her study got either one conditioning session or four of them. The sessions involved a flashing green light followed by a mild, non-painful electric shock to the ankle, a flashing yellow light with a lightly painful shock, or a flashing red light and a painful shock. After the participants had been conditioned to associate the different colours with pain, mild pain or a lack of pain, Colloca switched things around. Participants received mild shocks following flashing lights of all three colours. But that is not what the patients felt. After a red light flashed, they felt a painful shock. This is because they had been conditioned to associate a red light with a painful shock and a green light with a mild shock.

These conditioning studies show how open-label placebos probably work. When you go to see your doctor, the receptionist asks you to wait for him or her. Your doctor studied hard for years to become someone important enough that it is worth your while waiting until they are free to see you. When you make it into your doctor's office, it is very clean and sometimes full of impressive-looking medical instruments. Your doctor may even wear a white coat and probably a stethoscope. You are given a pill or an injection, and you get better.

Whenever you went to the doctor, you repeated the same procedure. Sometimes the treatment makes you better, and sometimes you would have got better on your own. That doesn't matter. What matters is that you learn to associate a visit to a doctor with getting better, much like Pavlov's dogs learned to salivate when they heard the bell they had been taught to associate with food. After a few successful doctor visits, the mere act of visiting the doctor can induce relaxation, boost the immune system and help you recover even without a pill. When I first learned about conditioning, I did not understand the difference between conditioning and expectancy, and many people I tell about it now ask me to explain the difference.

Much ado about nothing important

Academics get paid to make big deals out of simple things. Dozens of articles are published every year on the complexities of the difference between expectancy (from the last chapter) and conditioning (from this chapter). In fact, the difference is pretty simple. Both involve anticipating that something good will happen.

Expectancy occurs when someone *consciously* expects a positive reward, as when a trusted doctor says you are taking a powerful medicine that will make you feel much better very soon. This can help you get better, because expecting something good activates parts of your brain that induce your body to create its own drugs like dopamine.

Conditioning, on the other hand, is when you *subconsciously* expect a positive reward. After visiting the doctor many times and getting better, your body might become conditioned to expect a positive reward and react accordingly even before the doctor has a chance to say or do anything. Depending on what the placebo is, your individual characteristics, and what you are suffering from, either expectancy or conditioning, could be more important. More often than not, both come into play.

Takeaway: Reward and recondition yourself

My experience at the hands of a high-school basketball coach described earlier, and Luana Colloca's flashing red-light study from this chapter, show that we can be conditioned to have both positive and negative reactions. Since conditioning is a subconscious process, it can be very difficult to influence. Subconscious thoughts are usually hidden from us, and hidden things are hard to identify, let alone change. People like self-help guru Anthony Robbins say we can change our subconscious patterns very quickly, and sometimes they are right. More often than not, it takes patience and persistence for new positive thoughts to trickle down into our core so that they become part of our subconscious. The following is something I have used and found helpful.

Give yourself positive rewards for your achievements. Whenever you do something good, give yourself a reward. It is best to do it immediately so that you teach your brain the connection. Here is a list of some of the rewards I give myself.

Achievement	Reward
Major	
Publishing major academic article	Weekend getaway
Complete five chapters of book	
Medium	
Submit paper	Massage
Publish blog or newsletter	
Reach additional 1,000 social media followers	
Small	
Complete draft of paper or chapter	Long gym session

When doing this exercise, it is important not to choose things that you have no control over. There is no point planning to give yourself a reward if the sun comes out, because you have no control over the weather. Also, while it is great to dream big (even dream very big) it is also important to break it down into realistic steps. If your goal is to win a 100-metre Olympic gold medal and you are not a runner, give yourself smaller rewards for benchmarks along the way. For example, give yourself a reward for joining a running club and training with them regularly for three weeks.

PART IV

Individual Health Depends on Relationships

Ye cannot live for yourselves; a thousand fibres connect you with your fellow men, and along those fibres, as along sympathetic threads, run your actions as causes, and return to you as effects.

The Reverend Henry Melville,
Canon of St Paul's Cathedral

Beyond the intimate connection between mind and body health, we cannot separate our individual health from our connections with other people. In 1948, the World Health Organization (WHO) defined health as 'the state of complete physical, mental, and social wellbeing and not merely the absence of disease'. The definition has been controversial from the beginning, with some hailing it as positively revolutionary, and others saying it was vague and impossible to attain (who is completely healthy, according to this definition?).

Yet over the last several decades, a lot of evidence has shown that people who have good friends, family, and belong to social groups live an average of five years longer than those who do not. Social connections can also make us live better. In her bestselling book *The Village Effect*, Susan Pinker reports evidence that people who are isolated take longer to recover from sickness, feel stress more, are more prone to get heart attacks, get more complications when they get ill, and are more likely to get cancer. She warns that Internet culture threatens to worsen our health by isolating us from each other. The relationship between our individual health and our relationships with others extends further, with new studies showing that we become healthier when we do volunteer work. It also applies to healthcare relationships, with my systematic review showing that doctors can reduce pain as much as blockbuster drugs when they are allowed the time to express their empathy. I discuss this study in more detail in the next chapter on the doctor as a cure . . .

10

The Doctor Is a Cure

*Stephen Maturin [made] his medicines more revolting in
taste, smell and texture than any others in the fleet; and he
found it answered – his hardy patients knew with their
entire beings that they were being physicked.*

Patrick O'Brian, English novelist

The story of Quesalid

A hundred years ago, a boy named Maxugalis lived on what
is now called Vancouver Island in Canada. He became interested in Shamanism because he thought it was a sham, and
he wanted to expose their tricks to his community. The
problem was that he did not know how their tricks worked.
So he asked master shamans if he could sign up as an appren-
tice. Finally, one master shaman agreed. One day a patient
came to the shaman suffering from wild hysteria. The shaman
held the patient down and appeared to suck out a demon
from the patient's kidney into his mouth, then spat out a
bloody clump. However, Maxugalis had been watching carefully and he saw that the shaman had hidden some eagle
feathers between his lip and gum, which he had covered in
blood by sucking on his gum very hard. This was what he
then spat out. Curiously, however, despite this being a trick,
the patient appeared to get better.

With proof of the deception, Maxugalis prepared to expose
shamans as phonies. But before he did so, he wanted to
complete his apprenticeship, which required that he treat some
patients himself. Eventually a chief in a nearby village whose
grandson was very ill summoned him. On Maxugalis's arrival,
the chief looked at him and said, 'I dreamed of you as our
saviour'. Maxugalis was surprised – how could the chief

dream of a phoney shaman as a saviour? He did the eagle-feather trick, and was shocked when the chief's grandson recovered. The chief was so happy that he anointed Maxugalis with a new powerful shamanic name, 'Quesalid'.

Quesalid did not believe he was doing real medicine, but he saw that the rituals he used had a great effect on his patients. He went on to become one of the most successful and popular shamans in the region. According to anthropologist Claude Lévi-Strauss, 'Quesalid did not become a great shaman because he cured his patients; he cured his patients because he had become a great shaman.' In a nutshell, the patients got better because they believed in Quesalid's power.

What doctors did before drugs

Before the dawn of modern medicine, many treatments used by doctors, such as bloodletting, leeching and purging, were almost always ineffective and often harmful. Since they could not cure many illnesses, they had to focus on caring for the patient and communicating empathy. This became known as a 'bedside manner'. Doctors also encouraged their patients to take exercise and avoid overeating to *prevent* illness. It has been known from at least as far back as Ancient Greece that overeating and lack of exercise cause a large proportion of diseases. Hippocrates even claimed that excess eating caused more diseases than undereating.

Modern medicine changed things dramatically. We now have many powerful treatments ranging from anaesthetics that can knock you out, the drug adrenaline that can bring you back to life, surgery to fix damaged hearts, and antibiotics to cure deadly sepsis. Compared with these awesome treatments, Quesalid's tricks and bedside manner seem primitive. There is also less money in it.

You may not be surprised that the health benefits of empathetic communication with patients are not widely known. Expensive drugs and medical devices are aggressively promoted through sophisticated advertising, marketing and public relations operations funded by the pharmaceutical and medical supply companies. Careful listening, kindness, reassurance and sympathy cannot be patented. And – until recently – the benefits of these things have not been quantified, so it has been difficult to predict their financial benefits.

This all means that the doctor's role as a caring healer has been obscured beneath financial and bureaucratic systems that focus on targets and paperwork and all but ignore doctors' role as healers. General practitioners in England, for example, are often allotted a maximum of just ten minutes per patient. Patients complain about this. I did a study looking at how empathetic patients believe their healthcare practitioners (doctors, nurses or therapists) are. The results varied widely. We found sixty-four studies with approximately 5,000 patients across thirteen countries including the UK, Australia, the US, France, Germany and China. Male healthcare practitioners were not ranked as highly as female practitioners, and practitioners in Australia, the US, and the UK were considered to be more empathetic than their colleagues in other countries such as Germany and China. Empathetic care is not universally valued or applied, and this needs to change.

Patients are not the only ones who lose by the lack of focus on empathy: doctors suffer, too. Patients complain less about doctors who communicate well (which saves everyone involved a headache), and there is emerging evidence that doctors who express empathy are less likely to get burned out and are healthier. As a society, we have come to view doctors less and less as healers and more and more as pill dispensers. According to the British Medical Association, some GPs are required to see as many as sixty patients per day. Then doctors have to report to these managers to tell them what tests and treatments they have given out to make sure that they haven't given too much or too little.

Under these conditions, it is hardly surprising that doctor burnout rates are worryingly high and many promising medical students either look for work abroad or choose to work for consulting firms rather than becoming doctors. If doctors were valued as *healers* – the way Quesalid was – then the time they spent with patients would be valued as much as the fancy tests and treatments they give. In fact, recent evidence shows that doctors' old-fashioned bedside manner *is* as powerful as drugs for some common ailments.

Doctor's attention for treating irritable bowel syndrome

Harvard professor Ted Kaptchuk and his team studied the doctor effect on patients with irritable bowel syndrome (IBS). Half of participants in his study had a *normal* interaction with their doctor lasting no more than five minutes, while the others received an *augmented* forty-five-minute interaction. In these longer consultations, the doctors asked detailed questions about symptoms, how their condition related to relationships and lifestyle, and how the patients understood their condition. The doctors were instructed to display empathy, use engaging body language, and say things like, 'I can understand how difficult IBS must be for you.' The doctors were also told to pause for twenty seconds of thoughtful silence while feeling a pulse or thinking about the best treatment plan.

After three weeks, they measured the IBS symptoms in both groups of patients. The reduction in symptoms in the patients with augmented care was over twenty per cent greater than the reduction in the *normal* interaction group. Kaptchuk's study is not the only one. Dozens of others – including one systematic review that I conducted – have established that practitioner empathy can help cure patients suffering from common ailments such as pain and anxiety. This doesn't usually mean that empathy should replace medicine, but that it should be used alongside it.

When the doctor is the best medicine

Archie Cochrane, the pioneering Scottish doctor mentioned in Chapter One tells a dramatic and revealing story about his experience as a doctor in a POW camp during the Second World War:

> The Germans dumped a young Soviet prisoner in my ward late one night. The ward was full, so I put him in my room as he was moribund and screaming and I did not want to wake the ward. I examined him. He had obvious gross bilateral cavitations and severe pleural rub. I thought the latter was the cause of the pain and screaming. I had no morphia, just aspirin, which had no effect. I felt desperate. I knew very little Russian then and there was no one in the ward who did. I finally sat down instinctively on the bed and took him in my arms, and the screaming stopped almost at once. He died peacefully in my arms a few hours later. It was not the pleurisy that caused the screaming, but loneliness. It was a wonderful education about the care of the dying. I was ashamed of my misdiagnosis and kept the story secret.

Besides his brutal honesty, the interesting thing about Cochrane's story is that if morphine had been available, he would have given it to the patient. The morphine may have stopped the screaming, but it was not what the patient needed.

My colleague Karen Quinn (name changed to preserve anonymity) told me a less dramatic but perhaps more common story about three Oxford medical students who were told to diagnose a woman complaining of moderate shoulder pain. Let's call the woman Jane (again, name changed for anonymity). After twenty minutes of questioning, the students had a meeting. They wrote seven pages of notes and recommended three different drugs, including a powerful steroid injection. Karen examined the notes and did not see anything wrong – the students had followed the guidelines perfectly. But something told her there was more to the story. She went to see Jane and asked in a warm way how her family was. The patient immediately broke down in tears and told her about a recent tragedy involving her daughter. Jane did not need three drugs, she needed some tender loving care.

Palliative care versus aggressive treatment for end-of-life care

In his wonderful book *Being Mortal*, the American surgeon and writer Atul Gawande tells us the story of a man he met when he was a young intern. He calls the man Joseph Lazaroff. He was a city administrator who had lost his wife to lung cancer a few years earlier. He was now in his sixties and suffering from a widely metastatic prostate cancer, which is currently incurable. He had lost over fifty pounds, his abdomen, scrotum and legs had filled with fluid, he could not move his right leg, and he could not control his bowels. Gawande met Lazaroff as an intern on the neurosurgical team and discovered that it was even worse: the cancer had spread to his spine, where it was compressing his spinal cord.

Although the cancer could not be cured, they hoped it could be treated with radiation. They tried radiation, but it didn't help. So the head neurosurgeon offered him two options: comfort care or surgery to remove the growing tumour from his spine. Lazaroff chose surgery. Gawande's job, as the intern on the neurosurgery service, was to get Lazaroff's written confirmation that he understood the risks of the operation.

Gawande had recently graduated, so was inexperienced and very nervous. He was sweating as he tried to think of how to explain the risks of the invasive and risky surgery. In the best case, the operation would halt the progression of his spinal cord damage. It would not cure him, or reverse the paralysis. And no matter what they did, Lazaroff had at most a few months to live. Worse, the surgery was very risky. Surgeons would open his chest, remove a rib, and then collapse a lung to get at his spine, where they would try to cut out the tumour. He would lose a lot of blood and it would be hard to recover. Because he was already weak, there was also a high risk of serious complications like more paralysis, stroke, or even death. Apparently the neurosurgeon had described these dangers, yet Lazaroff was adamant that he wanted the operation. All Gawande had to do was go in to take care of the formal paperwork. He walked in to find Lazaroff looking grey and emaciated. He told him of the risks again. Lazaroff remained clear.

'Don't you give up on me,' he said. 'You give me every chance I've got.'

They did the surgery, which lasted almost nine hours. The surgeons rebuilt the spine with acrylic cement. The pressure was removed from the spine so the surgery was a 'success', but that was the only good thing about the story. In intensive care, Lazaroff developed respiratory failure, an infection and bleeding. After a few days, they finally had to admit he was dying. After two weeks, his son told the team to take Lazaroff off life-support, which they did. Lazaroff died.

Gawande believes that Lazaroff had chosen badly because the operation could not possibly have given him back his continence or anything close to the life he previously enjoyed. Lazaroff, Gawande said, 'was pursuing little more than a fantasy at the risk of a prolonged and terrible death – which was precisely what he got.'

Sadly, Lazaroff's story is not the exception. I accompanied my mother to hospital when she had metastatic cancer in her breasts, lungs, heart and bones, and the doctors told her she would recover quite a bit and be okay for a few years. This was not true, but to the doctors the important thing was prolonging life, not quality of life. In fact, the obsession with carrying out tests was to the exclusion of what we might call common-sense good care. Sometimes she had to wait as much as eight to ten hours when she had an appointment. Far from getting better after having her brain radiated and being put on numerous different pills, she ended up bedridden. Luckily, she realised what was happening and chose to stop the aggressive treatments. She died at home surrounded by loving family.

Often when people get a serious illness, the sad truth is there is no cure. So the important thing is to communicate with them lovingly to help them make difficult, but good, decisions, then give them loving care for the last weeks or months of their lives. Instead of this, according to Gawande, the medical profession is obsessed with giving heroic treatments such as multiple bouts of chemotherapy, aggressive surgery, and sticking tubes into people. These things rarely extend life, and almost always lower the quality of the remaining time people have to live. And instead of dying at home in the company of loved ones, many people die in hospitals hooked up to machines and so overmedicated that they have no clue what is happening.

To be sure, there are no easy answers to the decisions that Joseph Lazaroff and my mother had to make. Talking about fast-approaching death is even hard to imagine for most of us. But we can do better. There is another way that is not considered seriously enough: hospice care. Hospices were traditionally Roman Catholic institutions that provided hospitality for the sick, wounded or dying, as well as travellers or pilgrims. That is how they got their name. They are places people go when they accept that their illness cannot be cured and they are definitely going to die. Hospices provide round-the-clock expert care and support. People can also receive hospice care at home, through regular visits from nurses, and also have a 24/7 telephone service allowing them to summon help. This form of care focuses on treating symptoms like pain, fatigue and breathlessness, and on creating a warm, welcoming environment. It seeks to maximise patient independence as well as offering counselling and emotional support.

When Lazaroff said, 'Don't you give up on me', he was clearly stating that he did not want the option of hospice care. However, Gawande believes that he was never really offered it as a genuine choice, because nobody was prepared or skilled enough to have a difficult conversation with him. Palliative care doctors such as Dr Susan Block specialise in these end-of-life discussions. Block asks very sick patients questions such as:

- What do you understand about your illness and what it is likely to do to you?
- What are your concerns about what lies ahead?
- What kinds of trade-offs are you willing to make?
- How do you want to spend your time if your health worsens?
- Who do you want to make decisions for you if you can't?

These questions are not easy, because they raise difficult issues about the reality of serious disease. Block notes correctly that end-of-life discussions with patients and their families require no less skill than performing a complex surgical operation.

So why aren't patients like Lazaroff and my mother given the choice of palliative care? Besides the reason that some patients are desperate and will try anything, palliative care as a profession is not as sexy as surgery, oncology or intensive care, so the number of palliative-care doctors has been dwindling. Another reason is that by admitting that the patient is going to die, it can appear as though they are giving up. Fortunately, insurance companies are pushing for more palliative care, although their motivation is not concern for patients. Twenty-five per cent of healthcare funds are spent on the five per cent of people in their last year of life.

An insurance company called Aetna noted the disproportionate amount of money they were spending on the last few months of people's lives. They sponsored a trial where they offered 151 patients two choices. Either do as Lazaroff did and continue with their regular treatment regimes, or choose hospice care. Aetna paid for whatever option the patient chose. Since many patients are like Lazaroff and do not like the idea of giving up, Aetna allowed those who chose hospice care to continue with any treatment they liked. Since patients had the choice and since Aetna paid no matter what they chose, the patients had nothing to lose when they opted for hospice care.

Here is what happened. After skilled palliative-care doctors had the difficult conversation with the patients and they were able to see the options clearly, many chose hospice care. When I started reading this study, I was sure that those who chose hospice care would end up enjoying a better quality of life, but would die sooner. I was wrong.

Patients who chose hospice care ended up using emergency rooms half as much, intensive-care units only a third as much, and overall costs fell by one quarter. They were also able to prepare for their eventual demise, make final visits to favourite places, and talk to their grandchildren – things that those who opted for conventional treatment paths often were not able to do, because they ended up in intensive-care units.

The Aetna study is not unique. In another study, patients with terminal cancer who had discussions with palliative-care doctors about end-of-life goals were less likely to undergo cardiopulmonary resuscitation (CPR), be put on a ventilator or end up in an intensive-care unit. Most of them enrolled in hospices. They suffered less, were more physically mobile, and were able to interact with family – and from the time of their end-of-life discussions they lived twenty-five per cent longer than those who did not have them.

I witnessed the benefits of palliative care when my paternal grandmother became very ill with a serious digestive problem and had to have large chunks of her intestine removed. She was taking over twenty pills per day and was bedridden in hospital. She lost her appetite, and could barely swallow food without the help of a tube. She was already a small woman, but within a few months she dwindled away to a stick figure. She was very proud, and hated the indignity of being fed through a tube and having doctors poke and prod her before she had the chance to put some powder on her face.

Noting her distress, her four children consulted and decided to tell the senior doctor that it was time to stop trying to keep her alive with all these pills and tubes. They decided the best thing was to take her home and give her some peace and dignity. If the price was that Grandma would pass away, they had reconciled themselves to her dying sooner. The doctor tried to persuade them otherwise, saying that Grandma would not live more than a few weeks. 'At the most', the doctor said, 'she will live two more months.' But her children knew she hated the hospital and my father is very stubborn, so he ignored the doctor's recommendation and took her home.

They then hired a palliative-care nurse to take care of her at home for her final weeks. Two months passed, and she was far from dead. Instead, she had gained twenty pounds and had cravings for different kinds of food (especially McDonald's). She became close friends with the nurse, and lived on for two years with a much better quality of life than she would have enjoyed in hospital. For my grandmother, Lazaroff, and many others, palliative hospice care often improves quality of life, extends life, and costs less. Yet in order to provide it as a viable option, we need more doctors like Susan Block, who are as good at having conversations with patients about end-of-life choices as surgeons are with scalpels.

Unfortunately, as noted earlier, palliative care as a speciality seems to be shrinking, with doctors choosing more lucrative and prestigious options. Unless this changes, the problem remains that medicine focuses on treating and curing even in situations in which there are no effective treatments and there is no cure. 'In other words,' Gawande concludes, 'our decision-making in medicine has failed so spectacularly that we have reached the point of actively inflicting harm on patients rather than confronting the subject of mortality.'

Besides the benefit of taking them off aggressive treatments, how did a caring nurse help my grandmother? What was it about Cochrane's hug that helped the Russian soldier to stop

175

screaming? And how could Dr Quinn's gentle questioning cure Jane's painful shoulder? There are three possible explanations.

How the doctor effect works

The first way that empathetic doctors can generate better outcomes is by getting patients to give more accurate information. Some illnesses have embarrassing symptoms like diarrhoea, vomiting, funny smells and venereal problems. Sharing these symptoms can be difficult and uncomfortable. For some people, admitting that they have tried alternative cures is embarrassing. A doctor colleague once told me a story about a female patient whom he saw with advanced thyroid cancer. The disease was so advanced there was not much that could be done for her.

My colleague asked the patient why she did not visit earlier, when they might have had a chance to do something. The woman answered that she had used Reiki to treat some symptoms many years before, when the cancer first appeared. She had told her previous doctor at that time, but the doctor laughed and said Reiki healing was crap. The patient was angry and afraid to see any 'Western' doctor again. Whether or not you think Reiki is crap, unless the doctor empathises with the patient and is kind, the patient might well run away from the best available care.

Another way empathetic doctors can improve outcomes is by reducing the patient's anxiety. We saw in earlier chapters that too much anxiety and stress are bad for us. Empathetic doctors who make us feel that they care about us can help reduce our anxiety and stress. My colleague Professor Paul Little at the University of Southampton recently did a trial in which he proved this. He trained some doctors in a technique he called KEPe Warm. The technique involved:

- getting doctors to sit down when the patient was talking
- not interrupting patients

- taking patients' values into consideration
- verbally warming up throughout the consultation

Professor Little then compared the outcomes of almost 100 patients treated by doctors trained in KEPe Warm with almost 100 patients who saw doctors that did not use the technique. Those in the KEPe Warm group experienced an average reduction in anxiety of twenty per cent greater than those in the control group.

The third way empathetic doctors improve outcomes is by helping to boost the immune system. Being with a trusted doctor can send a powerful message to the body that it is okay to relax and jump start a full immune response. The immune system uses up a lot of energy. When you are sick and feeling tired, it is not only the disease that makes you feel unwell, it is also because your body is working hard to fight the illness. Because it takes up so much energy, it is not always in your survival interest to evoke a full immune response. If a caveman has an infection, but is alone, it might be dangerous to divert energy to his immune system, which will make him feel tired and cause him pain. If a wild animal or member of a hostile tribe attacks him in this state, he will not be able to defend himself. He might have a better chance of surviving if his body ignores the infection until he reaches the safety of his tribe. Then, once in a tent in his village, surrounded by trusted friends, it will be safe to invoke a full immune response.

Today wild animals are comparatively rare and most of us do not live in tribes, but the same evolutionary mechanisms are at work. When someone is ill and they feel they are being cared for by a trustworthy and reliable doctor, the body gets a message that it is okay for the immune system to operate at full capacity. Most of us have experienced this without necessarily knowing it. While doing exams, preparing to do a driving test, or something else we consider important, subconscious evolutionary mechanisms kick in to avoid the triggering of a full immune response to illness. This allows us to temporarily stave off tiredness and perform until the task at hand is over, at which point we crash and get ill for a few days, because we feel it is safe to do so. The empathetic doctor can make us feel safe and thus trigger the immune system to kick in and do its work.

Reversal: Negative doctors can harm

Just as negative expectations harm, so can unempathetic doctors. Karoline Vangronsveld is a psychologist in Sweden. She did an experiment in which she trained doctors to communicate with back-pain patients in one of two ways. One group were instructed to look at patients, nod to show they were listening, smiling, and say things like 'that must have been hard'. Those in the other group were told to glance down at papers while their patients were talking, ignore the patients' feelings, change the topic, or say things like 'not many people report that'. Patients' pain was reduced more in those seen by the empathetic doctors than those seen by the unempathetic group. These studies show that the words doctors use and the way they treat patients can have positive or negative effects.

Modern medicine as a ritual

The rituals, rites and quack treatments of ancient shamans like Quesalid seem primitive and even funny to many of us. Doctors these days do not use eagle-feather tricks to remove demons out of people's bodies. Today's doctors have real treatments, good surgical techniques, and high-tech diagnostic imaging devices that are much more effective than the shaman's potions and herbs. Medical doctors do not learn how to trick us, they are trained rigorously in medical science from accredited universities. They prove this with diplomas on their walls. It would be crazy to say that today's doctors are modern versions of Quesalid.

But it would be just as crazy not to notice the similarities. Some historians claim that modern medicine is just as ritualistic as ancient shamanism. What happens in today's hospitals is, after all, as mysterious to most of us as shamans were to our ancestors. Most of us do not understand how drugs or complex medical devices work, and we don't understand the language doctors use either, whether they are using the Latin terms, scientific jargon, or even the plain English equivalent. They use *hypertension* when they mean high blood pressure, *cardiovascular disease* when they mean heart problems, *upper respiratory tract infection* when they mean a cold, *syncope* when they mean fainting, and *epistaxis* is merely a nosebleed.

Often the language doctors use is further obscured by acronyms (*ENT* for *ear, nose and throat*, *MDD* for *major depressive disorder*, and *Rx* for *prescriptions*). Today's obscure medical language, fancy tests and doctor's diplomas may have a similar effect on our psyches as the shaman's feathers, rituals and rites. They both make the patient feel that their problems are being taken care of by someone powerful. Does this mean that we should give up on modern medicine and fly to the Brazilian rainforest to find a shaman next time we feel under the weather? No. But you can choose a doctor who will enhance the benefits of modern medicine with their empathetic bedside manner. And, as we'll see in the next two chapters, besides reaching out to the right kind of doctor, you will be healthier if you seek and maintain strong connections with friends, family and social networks.

Conclusion: Moving forward to the past

One of the main tools of modern medical research, the systematic review of randomised trials, is revealing that empathetic and positive communication has the same scientific backing as the latest tests and treatments for many common ailments. Many doctors already harness the healing power of their communication, and some might need a bit of reminding.

Takeaway: Choose the right doctor/healer

If you are a patient, choose a doctor who knows about evidence, *and* who is empathetic. Someone you feel understands your circumstances and values, and who you can see cares about you. If you do not have an empathetic doctor, you are missing out on the healing benefits of empathetic care and you should consider changing doctors. This does not mean you should choose a friendly idiot who can pat you on the back yet knows nothing about evidence. It also doesn't mean you should choose a doctor who always tells you what you want to hear.

For example, if your competent doctor is sure that you only have a cold and says that you do not need antibiotics, well maybe you don't, and you should listen. Fortunately, many doctors are both compassionate and familiar with the science of medicine. Finding a compassionate doctor who can communicate well is especially important if you or a loved one are facing the possibility of palliative care or further treatment. It can sometimes be uncomfortable to change doctors, however your health is at stake and the effort is worthwhile.

I I

Love as a Drug

Although living alone can offer conveniences . . . physical health is not among them.
     Julianne Holt-Lundstad, Professor of Psychology and
            Neuroscience at Brigham Young University

Dying of a broken heart?

North Dakota residents Clifford and Eva Vevea were happily married for sixty-five years, and in 2013 they died within a few hours of each other. That same year Illinois residents Robert and Nora Viands who had been married for seventy-one years died on the same day. A year earlier in the United Kingdom, Marcus Ringrose died twenty-four hours after his wife's funeral. Stories like this are reported in newspapers with sensational headlines like, 'You Really Can Die of a Broken Heart'. This is an exaggeration, because broken hearts rarely actually kill us. Yet research is beginning to prove there is some truth beneath the overblown headlines. Of course, poets have known for millennia that bad relationships are bad for our health. Shakespeare's Lady Montague dies of a broken heart after her son is banished in *Romeo and Juliet*. The Bible (Psalm 69) affirms that broken hearts can make people weak. Perhaps the great Persian poet Rudaki put it most romantically:

> *Look at the cloud, how it cries like a grieving man*
> *Thunder moans like a lover with a broken heart.*

Recently, scientists have found a growing body of evidence of real changes in the body following heartbreak. Broken Heart Syndrome, or Takotsubo cardiomyopathy to geeks like me, is an officially recognised medical condition. A Harvard study involving over 12,000 people found that married couples often die within a few months of each other. Another study at the Mayo Clinic found that people who were stressed out after the loss of a loved one were more likely to die sooner than those who were not. These results have been generalised in numerous studies.

You can die young of loneliness

A recent review of previous studies involving almost 50,000 people provides more evidence that loneliness is bad for our health. The study found out how isolated people were by asking things such as:

- Do you live alone or with other people?
- How much contact do you have with friends and family and other groups?
- Do you feel isolated or alone?

The results were clear. Seven years after first questioning the participants, lonely people were twenty-five per cent more likely to have died than those who were not lonely. In one of the studies that was included in the review, a group of researchers led by Carla Perissinotto in San Francisco followed 1,604 adults for six years between 2002 and 2008. They asked these patients if they (1) felt left out, (2) felt isolated, or (3) lacked companionship. They were then categorised as not lonely if they responded 'hardly ever' to all three questions and lonely if they responded 'some of the time' or 'often' to any of the three questions.

Lonely subjects were over ten per cent more likely to experience decline in the number of daily activities they could do, had more problems with their movements, and had more difficulty climbing stairs. Most strikingly, lonely people were more likely to die during the study. Some 22.8 per cent of the lonely people died over the six years compared with 14.2 per cent of those who were not lonely.

Another study involving more than 300,000 people showed that good social relationships can increase lifespan. At the beginning of the study, participants were asked about how many close family members and friends they had and what support they felt these provided. They then followed these people for many years. The results were clear: those with good social support lived an average of five years longer. Five years is a long time. It is as *good* as smoking is *bad*.

Why is loneliness bad for health?

One reason loneliness can be bad for health is that when people are isolated they are more likely to do things that are bad for health such as smoke, avoid exercise and sleep poorly. You may know of friends who tend to isolate themselves and start doing things that are bad for their health when they are having a tough time. One of my friends is a former professional sportsman. He was a very healthy and strong guy. When he split up with his long-term girlfriend, the group of friends of which I am part did not see him for a few weeks and he would not answer his phone. Together with two of his friends, we went to see him and there were pizza boxes all over the floor, the television was on, and he looked like he had not slept properly for days, because he hadn't. He had also started smoking.

We did not do any blood tests, but if we had, we would have noticed that his biology had changed. Poor sleep and lack of exercise can raise blood pressure and reduce immune function. We told him to get up and come to the gym with us. He told us to go away. Fortunately, the two other friends who went to visit him are bouncers at a nightclub, with a lot of practice at making people get out of places when they decide it is the right time for them to go. So we dragged him to the gym and made him do a workout, then took him out for dinner. We put the pizza boxes in a rubbish bag and did a quick clean of his place. One of us visited him every day to drag him to the gym and make sure he did not smoke. Within about three weeks, he was more or less back on his feet.

This was a success story that was made possible by a good network of friends. Unfortunately, evidence suggests that we have fewer and fewer close friends.

Is loneliness an epidemic?

In the 1950s, over eighty per cent of doctors and most of the population smoked, because they did not know it was bad for their health. Of course, loneliness is not considered to be a good thing, but it is not the subject of public health information campaigns. Yet loneliness seems to reduce our lifespan by almost as much as smoking, and it is on the rise in developed nations. Our grandparents' and even parents' generation had to share rooms, cars (if they had one), and phones with other family members. Now most of us grow up with our own rooms, nearly everyone over the age of eighteen in North America has their own car, and nearly everyone over twelve has their own phone. My nephew is eight years old and complains that 'everyone in his class' has their own mobile phone. He may be exaggerating, but it is certainly true that some eight-year-olds have their own mobiles.

While there are certainly benefits to mobile-phone and other technology, it is associated with wider changes that have led to less intergenerational living, greater social mobility, bigger houses, delayed marriage, and increased divorce. As a result, we have become more socially fragmented and therefore more isolated. Compared with twenty years ago, three times more Americans report having nobody to confide in. One in ten people in the UK report feeling lonely often, a third have a close friend or relative whom they think is very lonely, and half think that people are getting lonelier.

Technology and wealth are neither bad nor good in themselves. The problem is that together they make it easy for us to be lazy and lonely. We need to use wisdom and intelligence so that our technology and wealth benefit us. I called Professor Sheldon Cohen, who did much of the research quoted in this chapter, to ask him why he never took up any job offers away from his native Pittsburgh. He said he refused, partly so that he and his family can maintain their strong social ties in the city where they grew up.

My former rowing coach, Dusan Kovacevic, did something more dramatic. He went to Canada to get away from the Balkan War in the mid-1990s. Within a few years, he achieved what many Serbs dreamed of – Canadian citizenship. Yet soon after he received his Canadian passport, he returned to Belgrade. There, he lived in his small apartment in the suburbs and took a prestigious but modestly paying (and politically difficult) job as a rowing coach at his former club. He also had to deal on a daily basis with his extended family every day. This is great in some ways because they help with babysitting, but it has a big downside too.

As any of you with large families will know, some drama is inevitable. In Dusan's case, his mother is lovely and supportive, yet also completely domineering. She also lives next door. Apparently, she comes from an area that is so cold in the winter that cars could not reach it between December and April. The people in that area have a strong work ethic, partly because in winter those who are inactive risk being frozen to death. Under these circumstances some people from this region don't have time for jokes or trivial arguments. For Dusan's mother, trivial things include arguing about who is right and wrong. She knows she is right.

Why did Dusan move from Canada back to what is clearly a materially poorer and more complicated family life? His friends did not understand and thought he was crazy. When I asked him to explain, he said, 'In Ancient Greece, the most serious punishment was exile, even more serious than death. In Canada, I felt as if I was exiled from my family and friends. In Canada, everyone is rich, but you have to make an appointment to see them. In Belgrade, people just walk in without any appointment.'

I have been to visit him, and what he says is true. His in-laws, sister and mother drop in frequently without invitation or warning. His children share one room. His mother tells him what to do (he doesn't listen). In the midst of all that chaos, he is happier than when he was in Canada, despite the prospects of a bigger house, a bigger car, more money, and much more security. As Julianne Holt-Lunstad, the psychologist who led the large review of loneliness and health, put it: 'Although living alone can offer conveniences . . . physical health is not among them.'

How do social networks improve health?

The main reason social *isolation* is bad for health is that it removes the benefits of social *integration*. To prove more definitively that smoking caused lung cancer, researchers also had to show that *stopping* smoking reduced the risk of lung cancer (which it does). Julianne Holt-Lunstad did the same thing to check how isolation was bad for health. She did a systematic review of studies that looked at the benefits of having friends, family, and belonging to social groups. She found 148 studies with 308,849 people and found that they lived an average of five years longer when they were well integrated into their social networks.

Benefits of the links to other people come in three categories. First, friends and family provide actual help. You might take a disabled friend for a walk, lend an ear to someone who is feeling sad about a bereavement, or inform a relative with an illness about a new treatment of which they have not heard. Researchers call this the *main effects hypothesis*. Second, helpful friends and family can make you feel protected and less anxious, thus reducing the harmful effects of stress – or the *stress buffering hypothesis*, if you want to get technical. Finally, human contact boosts the amount of a hormone called oxytocin in our bodies, which is good for us. I will say a bit about each of the explanations for how social networks improve health.

Friends point you in the right direction

In one of Sheldon Cohen's most interesting studies, he gave a group of people a virus that causes the common cold. He also asked them whether they:

1. were married
2. had a parent with whom they had contact
3. had a family member with whom they had contact
4. had a neighbour with whom they had contact
5. had a friend with whom they had contact
6. had a workmate with whom they had contact
7. had a schoolmate with whom they had contact
8. volunteered
9. were part of a wider group with or without religious affiliation

Cohen reported that participants who ticked at least six of the roles listed above were only *half* as likely to develop a cold in the days after being exposed to the cold virus, compared with those who were less socially integrated. This study and others like it have been replicated numerous times. Good social support can stop people getting certain diseases or reduce their symptoms. The reason the main effects hypothesis works is clear. Besides making us feel better, family and friends can help us through illnesses.

For example, someone might begin to develop a cold and feel tired because they have become infected with the cold virus, but they do not have a full-blown cold yet. A friend or family member might encourage them to take a rest, make them a cup of tea, or do something else that might boost their immune system and help them fight the cold more quickly. Someone who is knowledgeable about exercise and diet might help a friend lose weight or provide them with an individually tailored exercise programme. A family member might let you know about a website that contains advice on healthy eating. Having an extensive and caring social network increases the chances of you becoming aware of these opportunities.

I will give you a recent example from my own experience. A close friend had to go to the hospital recently for a minor operation on his ankle. He was meant to be out by noon. I drove him there, made sure he settled in properly, and told him about the benefits of listening to calming music for recovery after an operation. He followed this advice, but he was not ready to leave at noon. I had to get to London to give a speech, so I called another friend who went to the hospital to pick him up. The doctors told him not to walk for three days, so other friends brought him food. Now none of this caused any miracles, but three days after his operation he was up and walking around. It is easy to see that someone without the support of friends might have taken a few more days to recover.

I can remember a time that my friends helped me to stay healthy. In September 2014, my mother passed away in Montreal. Within twenty-four hours, my three best friends made their way from three different countries to support me. People are more likely to drink, smoke and eat junk food when a family member dies. I don't remember being tempted by any of these, but I was certainly not in my normal state of mind and if I had been around alcohol, cigarettes or junk food I don't know what I would have done. As it turns out, having supportive friends around kept me feeling better than I would have done otherwise. One of them actually dragged me on a two-and-a-half-hour run that helped me release stress and made me feel so tired that I had a great sleep, when normally the grief might have kept me awake.

You may even have an example from your own experience. If you are a parent, you could rightly worry that if your kids mix with people who smoke, drink or take drugs, they might also take up these habits. This is because being around people who make healthy choices makes it more likely that you will do so. Studies show that if you are a smoker and your friends quit smoking, you are more likely to quit too. You may also remember a time when the people around you helped *you* to make a healthy choice. So the studies I am describing here probably confirm what you already know from experience. However, social support does more than provide help: it also makes you feel generally calmer. That's the other reason why social support improves health: it protects us from the damaging effects of stress.

Social support protects against stress

In 1983 over 700 Swedish men aged fifty years and over were given physical health assessments. Researchers also handed the men questionnaires about:

- Whether they were experiencing stressful events in their lives, such as financial trouble, divorce, problems with the health of a family member.
- Whether their social networks were providing emotional support.

After seven years, forty-one of the men had died. When the investigators looked at the causes of death, they found the usual suspects such as cholesterol levels, obesity and heart disease had not been the major killers. Obese people with high cholesterol were as likely to die as slim people with normal cholesterol. However, those men who reported having lots of stress in their lives were three times more likely to die sooner than those who did not. This is not surprising given the mechanism of stress and the fight-or-flight response described in earlier chapters: stress changes your biology in measurable ways, and a lot of it does so in harmful ways.

When the researchers looked more closely at the men's questionnaire responses, they found the stressed-out men who had strong social support were just as healthy as the relaxed men. So stress only increased the chances of an early death in those without strong bonds with friends and family. Think back to stressful events in your own life and you might find this chimes with your experience. Having good people around does not simply provide assistance and advice; it makes you feel more relaxed and less anxious, because you feel supported. I certainly felt that way when my friends flew in after my mother passed away. This brings us to the third reason why better social networks improve health: contact with social networks also helps the body produce its own drug: oxytocin.

Oxytocin: the love drug

Oxytocin is rare among hormones in that it gets as much press as Hollywood celebrities. It even has a nickname: the cuddle hormone. It makes you want to connect with people, especially when there are problems, and it also reduces your stress. It can even make you empathetic when you see someone who looks like they are having a tough time. Some people say we should snort the stuff to become better people. In one study, people actually did snort the stuff.

A researcher invited thirty-seven healthy men to an experiment without telling them what was being studied. He then gave them either oxytocin or a placebo to snort. Then the researcher did his best to make these poor men very nervous by making them do three things that normally make people anxious and nervous. He told the men they would have to:

- Give a speech in front of an audience of three judges who would make audio and video recordings of their performance.
- Count backwards from 1,022, in increments of 13 with any mistakes being punished by them having to start again, also in front of an audience.
- Do a job interview in front of a panel with a conspicuous camera trained on them.

The men were given ten minutes to prepare. Half had to prepare alone, while the other half were allowed to bring their best friend along to offer support. The participants were divided into four groups: with a friend and given oxytocin, no friend and oxytocin, a friend and given a placebo, and no friend and given a placebo. Throughout the study, researchers measured the men's levels of the stress hormone cortisol. As the researchers expected, cortisol levels were highest in the group that did not bring their best friends and did not have oxytocin, and lowest in the group that had oxytocin and their best friends along. The study provides further proof that a lack of social interaction increases our stress levels.

Reversal: Just as social integration helps, negative social interaction can harm

If you choose a criminal gang as your social group, you will probably not live longer. It is not just any family, friends and social group that improve health, but the right ones. Less dramatic than joining a gang, Sheldon Cohen did another study proving the negative impact of toxic relationships on health. His team interviewed 276 adults to find out whether they were experiencing social conflicts, such as marital conflict lasting more than one month. They then exposed them to a common cold virus. They found that people who were experiencing chronic social stress were more than twice as likely to get an infection as those who were not stressed out.

When I talk to groups about the negative impact on health of damaging relationships, there is always one person in the room who tells me a story about someone in their close circle of friends or a family member whom they feel is toxic. Since no family or group of people is perfect, we probably all have some of these people in our lives. Those attending such discussions often ask me what to do. The truth is I don't know. And even if I did, the answer for one person in a particular set of circumstances would be different to that for someone else. I can only tell you what I do when this situation affects me: I reach out to a wise, trusted person in my social network to ask for their help. This works very well.

A note about proving causes

This section is a bit geeky, so if you are not interested in proving causes, skip to the next section. Here is the question: does social support cause better health, or does better health cause social support (remember the chicken-and-egg problem from Chapter Five)? Sick people do not have the capacity to keep up with friends or family as much as healthy people. So when we look at the studies that prove a connection between good social networks and healthier lives, how do we know which comes first?

Some of those who carried out this research were well aware of this problem, so they looked more carefully at how healthy participants were at the beginning of the studies. They wanted to see whether those with and without social networks were as healthy as each other before they took part in the research. Their conclusion was that it was the social networks that seemed to cause better health rather than vice versa.

In one Canadian study, researchers checked fifty-five initial health conditions ranging from heart disease, respiratory conditions, and mental-health conditions, such as dementia and depression. They also measured and controlled for forty-one additional miscellaneous conditions, ranging from electrolyte abnormalities to coeliac disease. They still found that those with stronger social support networks were more likely to have stayed healthy by the end of the study.

You might ask why the researchers did not simply do a randomised trial of people with the same initial health status to avoid having to rely on measuring fifty-five health conditions and doing fancy statistical analyses. For example, they might have chosen a thousand people, then flipped a coin to decide which ones would be allowed to have a strong social support network for the period of the study. This of course would be impossible, except perhaps in an extraordinarily authoritarian state. You cannot randomise people to have good friends and family or not. There are some other types of experiments, however, that lend more support to the view that social support improves health.

Some studies in the 1950s of foster homes came close to what we would consider to be a rigorous trial today. The homes were full of signs with instructions such as 'Wash your hands twice before entering this ward.' These places were often clean, but the atmosphere was cold and the foster children experienced little human warmth. Then psychologist Harold Skeels removed some children from a sterile orphanage with this kind of environment and handed them into the care of young women. The children's IQs rose dramatically. Other similar studies followed and eventually the World Health Organisation published a report that emphasised the importance of human contact and warmth for both the mental and physical health of those in foster care. Reading the report, one doctor in a foster home took down the 'Wash your hands twice' sign and replaced it with a sign saying, 'Do not enter this nursery without picking up a baby'. Even more dramatic experiments proved that social networks improve health in monkeys.

In the 1960s, scientists took baby monkeys from their mothers and kept them separated for periods of several weeks. The baby monkeys screamed, scratched and sucked on the wires of their cages in search of their mothers' breasts. They clung to the cage walls and eventually curled up into little balls and stopped moving. Many became ill and at least one died. In some of the experiments the baby monkeys were reunited with their mothers and became happy again. We do not have all the details of what happened in other experiments, in which they were not returned to their mother's care following separation.

This book is not about the thorny debate over animal rights.

But in this case, it is hard not to side with activists who pointed out that the experimenters were cruel to the monkeys and did not teach us anything new. We already knew from the foster children experiments that parental warmth was necessary for normal development. If you take baby humans and primates away from their mothers, they get mentally and physically ill.

If you add all this evidence up, we can safely conclude that the chicken or egg problem (at least for social networks) has been solved. It is fair to say that good social networks improve health rather than vice versa. You can, of course, study a lot more about proving causes than what I have written here. Philosophers have been studying causes for thousands of years and still cannot agree on whether they exist. However, hopefully you now have enough information to form an educated opinion about whether you agree with me that social networks improve health. You are also better equipped to make informed decisions about whether the causes of new discoveries and breakthroughs you might see featured in newspapers are exactly as they are reported or not.

Takeaway: Three ways to improve your health by improving your social networks

These are three things that are based on the systematic review evidence discussed in this chapter. You can use them to reduce mild to moderate depression, as well as boost your health and wellbeing. Your life will also be more fun.

1. **Join a group that interests you.** There are so many options, from hiking and singing, to playing chess and eating cheese. Most are free and easy to join so there is no need to be lonely. If you can find a group involving a cause you believe in, all the better. Martin Luther King Jr said that if you haven't found anything you are willing to die for, you are not fit to live. You don't need to be quite this

radical, but it is true that participating in a meaningful social group helps you reduce stress by giving you something bigger to focus on.

2. **Connect with a family member**. Invite them over for lunch, tea or dinner, or just give them a call. If you do not have any family members that you can connect with, then opt for a friend, or even someone from the group you are about to join after reading number 1 above! If you think about it, of course, we are all related if you go back far enough. We are all busy these days, so scheduling these meetings can be important.

   My colleague Iain Chalmers told me that he has lunch every Thursday with his three best friends. It is a regular event that is permanently in their diaries. I have regular weekly meetings with some friends, and my friend Colin even uses a spreadsheet. The spreadsheet contains a list of all his friends, and he circulates through the list. The sheet seems a bit robotic to me, but I always like it when I get a call from him so I can't complain. The reality is that unless we schedule things, we tend to put them off.

3. **Reach out to someone**. Do something this week for someone else, even if it is small. Smile and say hello to a homeless person. Reach out to a friend, family member or acquaintance who could use some social interaction. It will make the world a healthier and better place. And as we will see in the next chapter about oxytocin, you will be helping yourself as much as you help the other person.

12

In Giving We Receive

You can't help someone get up a hill without getting closer to the top yourself

General H. Norman Schwarzkopf, Jr

The total number of minds in the universe is one

Erwin Schrodinger,
Nobel prize-winning Austrian physicist

To give is more blessed than to receive

Melvyn Amrine, aged eighty-three, had been married to Doris for sixty years. They lived in Little Rock, Arkansas, and Melvyn had recently developed severe Alzheimer's. He also had trouble walking and he could not even remember marrying Doris. So when he disappeared on 10 May 2014 (the day before Mother's Day), Doris got extremely worried and called the police.

Officers Brian Grigsby and Troy Dillard soon found Melvyn two miles away from his home walking quickly. They asked him to get in their car to take him home, but Melvyn refused. They asked him a few questions. He could not remember his own name, he didn't know where he was, and he did not have his wallet or any form of identification. He knew only one thing: he needed to buy flowers for his wife for Mother's Day, just like he had done every year since they had their first child. Melvyn made it very clear to the police that 'he wasn't going home until he got those flowers'. The police were touched by his determination and took him to the flower shop on the way home. They helped him choose some cream-coloured roses. Sergeant Grigsby even secretly paid for the flowers because Melvyn had forgotten his money.

When they brought him home, Doris cried when she saw the flowers. She said, 'Even though the mind doesn't remember everything, the heart remembers.' Grigsby and Dillard were praised in the news, and felt great. They might also have made themselves healthier along the way.

Health benefits of volunteering

The flip side of helping someone is being helped ourselves. In 2011, Professor Daniel George in Pennsylvania did a randomised trial with thirty people who had dementia. Half of them volunteered for one hour per week with school children, helping them with reading, writing and history. The others did not do volunteer work. At the end of the study, stress was lowered more in those who volunteered than in those who did not. However, the study was small, so in 2013 researchers did a systematic review that combined four trials of volunteering. The studies were all quite different and had mostly positive but mixed results. Volunteering seemed to improve things like cognitive function, physical activity, strength, walking speed and stress. However, it did not seem to have an effect on number of falls, which is important for older people. Neither did it affect purpose in life or loneliness. The authors of the review concluded that more research was necessary.

More and more recent research is establishing a link between volunteering and health. In the most recent study I am aware of, fifty-two high-school students in Canada were randomised to volunteer once per week by helping younger students with their homework, sports, or other after-school activities. Another fifty-four students did not do any volunteer work. The researchers then took blood samples from both groups. They found that the students who volunteered lost more fat, lowered cholesterol more, and had better immune system function, compared with the students who did not volunteer.

One study found that merely thinking about others being helpful can be beneficial. Harvard psychologist David

McClelland asked one group of students to watch a film of Mother Teresa caring for orphans in Calcutta. He asked other students to watch a neutral film. After the viewings, he found those who had watched the Mother Teresa film had higher levels of an important protective immune system antibody called salivary immunoglobin A than those in the control group. Interestingly, this immune system boost occurred whether or not students agreed with Mother Teresa's religious beliefs. This trial suggests that having altruistic thoughts can improve health by strengthening the immune system.

How helping helps the helper

If you volunteer to take a dog for a walk, you are increasing your physical activity, which is good for your health. Any volunteering that connects you to people could help you reap the health benefits of social networks discussed in the previous chapter. It may also reduce stress and help us relax by taking our minds off our own problems. An evolutionary mechanism was even suggested by a US National Institute for Mental Health study in which nineteen volunteers were given money and a list of good causes to which they could donate.

Brain scans showed networks of brain cells that transmit dopamine between brain regions were activated in the people who donated money. As we saw in Part III, dopamine is the brain-messaging chemical that makes us feel good when we do something beneficial to our survival. Research showing that we get a dopamine high when we are altruistic suggests we have evolved that way because our ancestors were more likely to overcome the hardships they faced if they helped each other out.

Does the discovery of mirror neurons help explain how volunteering helps?

In the early 1990s, neuroscientist Giacomo Rizzolatti and colleagues at the University of Parma, Italy, discovered the existence of brain cells in laboratory monkeys. The cells were activated both when they performed actions and when they watched others doing so. He called these 'mirror neurons' and went on to show that humans have them too. Mirror neurons are located in the part of the brain called the premotor cortex. Neurons in the premotor cortex send messages that cause things like arm movement. The mirror neurons in our brain fire when we see someone else move. So if we see a person lift their arms, the neurons in our premotor cortex responsible for lifting our arms also fire. Our neurons rarely fire strongly enough to actually lift our arms, but sometimes they do.

For example, if you watch fans at an American football game, you can sometimes see them move their bodies when the quarterback makes a challenging pass. These motor neurons seem to be important for learning through imitation. I can learn how to drive by watching someone else drive. Athletes learn to improve their game by watching other athletes. Or they can improve through visualisation – which is imagining themselves doing what they would like to do as if they were someone else.

Besides mirror neurons that fire when others engage in movement and that can help us learn about movement, there are also mirror neurons for touch. We all know that being touched can trigger a variety of emotional responses, as can watching others touching. Why does watching a romantic film scene, or seeing the bride and groom kiss at a wedding, have us dabbing tears from our cheeks? Our brains are mirroring the experiences of the people we see in front of us.

The potential role of these mirror neurons in establishing

empathy, through a dissolving of the separation between individuals, has led neuroscientist V. S. Ramachandran to call them 'Gandhi Neurons'. So perhaps at the same time that we improve others by being kind, mirror neurons in us are activated that are beneficial.

Saying thank you makes you healthier

Just as volunteering benefits the volunteer, a similar number of studies show that expressing gratitude has health benefits. You probably remember your parents reminding you to say the magic words 'thank you' because it is considered to be polite. What they probably did not tell you is that being grateful can also make you healthier. In a series of studies, American psychologists randomised 400 adults, some of whom had neuromuscular disorders, to receive one of three treatments:

- Gratitude: participants were asked to list the things they had reasons to be grateful for in the last week.
- Hassles: participants were asked to list the unpleasant irritants or hassles that had occurred in the last week.
- Events (control): participants were asked to list the events that had occurred in the last week.

After the participants had been doing this for ten weeks, the investigators found those who had been listing their reasons to be grateful had improved more than the others in terms of their general outlook on life, physical symptoms of disease, and how refreshed they felt when they awoke. Focusing on being grateful seemed to make them feel better, less depressed, and also reduced the symptoms of some illnesses. Simply making a list of things for which we are grateful thus has a similar effect to some drugs.

Many other studies have similar results. In 2013, Lisa Bolier and her colleagues in the Netherlands did a systematic review of 'positive psychology', which I have mentioned in earlier chapters. Positive psychology encourages people to have a positive outlook on life. Instead of focusing on problems and negative things that have happened in the past, positive psychology teaches people to emphasise the good things in their lives. As part of that, it encourages them to be grateful for these good things, and to express that gratitude.

Bolier's review covered thirty-nine studies with a combined total of over 6,000 patients. Many positive psychology interventions had a beneficial effect on patients with depression and on their general wellbeing. However, the results were mixed, with some showing greater benefits than others. The more positive psychology that patients had, the greater the effects seemed to be. Also the results cannot be attributed to the benefits of gratitude alone, because positive psychology is much broader than that. However, gratitude is certainly an important part of these approaches.

So it seems that doing nice things for others, as well as being thankful for nice things others (or life) have done for us, can make us healthier. But something is fishy about this: isn't the aim of helping people to help them? If I help others in order to help myself, does that not mean I'm being selfish?

The possibility of altruism

Do we ever actually do something for others, or are all our motives selfish? This raises an old philosophical question about the possibility of altruism, with some saying that we never do things for others, but only for our own benefit (it makes us feel good). The first thing to say about this is that from the point of view of a starving person it doesn't matter. If someone helps them with food, the starving person might not care too much about the possibility of altruism, because they are just happy to receive food.

And against the philosophers who claim that altruism is impossible, there are some cases where it is hard to see how the person helping got any benefit. For example Mother

Teresa, gave up all material comforts to care for some of the sickest people in the world. Or during emergencies, some people put their own lives at risk to help others.

Wesley Autrey, also known as the Hero of Harlem, saved Cameron Hollopeter, in a way that put his own life at risk. Here is what happened. At lunch-time on 2 January 2007, Autrey was waiting for a train at the 137th Street subway station in Manhattan with his two young daughters. After having a seizure, Hollopeter stumbled and fell onto the tracks. As a bystander held his daughters back from the edge of the platform, Autrey dived onto the tracks. With the lights of an oncoming train getting brighter, he realised there was not enough time to lift Hollopeter up to the platform, so he threw himself over his body and held him down in a drainage trench between the tracks. Though the operator of the train applied the brakes, all but two cars still passed over them, close enough to touch his cap. Now it is true that Autrey got famous after the incident. However, at the time he performed the act, it is hard to see how he thought he was doing it to help himself.

Altruism confuses some biologists, too, because evolutionary theory has trouble explaining it. You might think it makes sense in evolutionary terms: one monkey turns its back to another monkey, and the other monkey will pick out parasites. Then they will change roles so that both monkeys get parasites removed from their backs. Both monkeys benefit from altruism. However, according to evolutionary theory, genes mutate randomly and the random mutations that increase the chances of survival and having children get passed on, and those that reduce the chances of survival do not. That means an altruism gene would have arisen randomly in just one monkey, and it is hard to see how that original altruistic gene would have been passed on.

The first human, or human ancestor, to randomly get an altruism gene was almost certainly at a disadvantage. He or she would pick parasites from another monkey's back. Then the now parasite-free monkey would wander off to find food or to find a partner to procreate with. Meanwhile the altruistic monkey would have more parasites (and more sickness as a result) and less time to reproduce or eat, because it was spending time picking parasites from other monkeys. So, the story goes, the altruistic gene would decrease the chances of survival and die out.

Evolutionary theorists show another thing that makes the altruism gene more likely to fail: it encourages the 'weaker' genes to survive, weakening the species. If a species does what Autrey did, and performed altruistic acts to help someone who otherwise would not remain alive, then the altruistic individual is helping weak genes to survive. Weakening the species reduces chances of survival in the long run, which again would suggest that a species that developed altruism genes would die out. These evolutionary stories about the origins of altruism are just speculation. The fact is that we do not know how altruism evolved, and evolutionary theory makes it difficult to see how it could have arisen on a wide scale in the first place.

Yet altruism is pervasive in nature in spite of the difficulties in explaining how it first evolved. Wolves and wild dogs bring back meat to pack members not present at the kill. Vervet monkeys scream to warn each other when a predator approaches, even though the screaming attracts the predator's attention to himself or herself. Mongooses support older, sick and injured animals. Many birds will help feed and raise the young of other birds. Termites will give themselves a fatal wound to release a sticky substance from a specialised gland so that invading ants get stuck.

The best evolutionary explanation for altruism, proposed by political scientist Robert Axelrod and evolutionary biologist W. D. Hamilton in 1981, is that we share genes with our close relatives, so helping our relatives will help our genes survive. If this is right, it means it is not our *individual genes* that fight selfishly for survival, but our *group*'s genes. It seems to fly in the face of the belief that we live in an individualist dog-eat-dog world, in which the best way to allow our species to thrive is to allow the fittest individuals and their genes to rise to the top, even if that causes those people at the bottom to starve.

Altruistic behaviour means helping the weak and their genes to survive, making the group weaker. But if the unit of evolution is not our individual genes, but our group's genes, then it is good to help one another. This idea offers an evolutionary underpinning to the evidence from the last chapter, which suggested that good relationships with family, friends and social groups make us live longer. Maybe that is why a study showed that helping others is more beneficial for our health when our motives are altruistic.

Researchers followed the experiences of over ten thousand Wisconsin high-school graduates from their graduation in 1957. In 2004, the graduates were asked:

- Whether they had volunteered in the past ten years
- How often they volunteered, and how long they volunteered for
- The reasons why they volunteered

Their reasons for doing voluntary work were then classified as selfish, such as self-exploration, looking to feel better, or to escape from troubles, or altruistic including feeling compassion for people in need, or community service. Like other studies, this one showed that people who volunteered more were healthier – in fact, they were less likely to die early. When the researchers looked deeper, they found that the health benefits of volunteering only went to those who did so for altruistic reasons.

The research on the benefits and importance of helping others reflects the teachings of many religions. Jesus said that giving is more blessed than receiving. The Torah requires that ten per cent of a Jew's income be allotted to righteous deeds or causes; Zakat, or helping the needy, is one of the five pillars of Islam. And charity work, known as Dana, is a virtue in both Hinduism and Buddhism.

Reversal: Helping is good, but some helping can be bad for you and the people you are trying to help

If you are helping others so much that you don't even take care of yourself, then your body and mind can become stressed and unhealthy. I witnessed this while watching my sisters raise their children. Like my mother, my sisters could not bear to hear a new-born baby cry. When their babies woke up, they woke up. This was empathetic; however, they ended up not sleeping and even becoming ill. As a result, they could not care for any of their children properly.

So they had to learn to let the babies cry sometimes, in order to get enough rest to be able to look after their children. This is kind of common sense. But as Voltaire said, 'Common sense is not so common.' Many of us do not do enough to help others, and I hope this chapter motivates you (as it has me) to lend a hand. But use common sense and don't suddenly start doing so much that you end up sick yourself.

Equally, doing the wrong sort of volunteering, perhaps where an individual stands the risk of verbal or physical abuse, can be detrimental. When my sister was a teenager, she could not walk past a homeless cat or dog or person and not try to help, which is great. However, she once stopped her car illegally on the highway to save a cat. She almost certainly saved the cat, but she also endangered her life.

A different kind of worry is that sometimes we think we are helping others, but we are harming them. I used to give money to homeless people (I still do at times). However, I got to know some of them and, at least in Oxford, the money is usually used for drugs rather than food. So now I offer to buy them a coffee, and they usually accept. This wrong kind of volunteering that might harm the people we are trying to help is apparently common in international volunteer work. An increase in people wanting to help in orphanages in Nepal led to a dramatic increase in the number of orphanages, some of which are involved in child trafficking. It also leads to some of the children feeling abandoned, because the volunteers do not stay long.

Karjit, a youth from Humla, who grew up in a series of children's homes in Kathmandu and Pokhara, despite not being an orphan, was interviewed and he complained:

> There were so many volunteers: short-time, long-time, middle-time, according to visa! . . . Sometimes they organise programme and I don't want to go. Children sometimes feel angry, because they want to do what they want. There is a nice movie and children they want to watch, but volunteers organise a football programme and house managers say you have to go. And all children were angry . . . Why foreigners come to Nepal? Why do they go in orphanage? That time they come for short time and they give love to us, but then they leave, and when I write they don't reply. I say to a volunteer, 'Sister, I am very lonely', and they say, 'No problem, I am here', but then they go their country and I write, but they don't reply. When I was little everyone can love me, now I am big and I need love.

Fortunately, cases like Karjit's are the exception rather than the rule, and there are a lot of things we can all do to help the world (and ourselves) without doing more harm than good.

Takeaway 1: Seven things you can do to help others and yourself

Okay, volunteering is good for us. But we are all busy, and how can we be sure that we are not accidentally doing harm, like the volunteers may have done to Karjit? There are good-news answers to both of those questions. First, volunteering a reasonable amount does not take time. In fact a study shows that it makes you feel like you have more time. This is probably because it makes you feel positive, relaxed, happy and energised. And you are right that it is impossible to know for sure whether something you do is really going to help, because we cannot see into the future. At the same time, there are at least seven things you *can* do that are almost certainly helpful for lowering your anxiety, improving your health, and helping someone else.

1. Do something nice for a family member. This could take many shapes or forms. You could take them out for lunch or dinner, or visit or send a card.
2. Help a colleague at work who is struggling with a task that you are an expert in.
3. Give your time to a charity (see guidelines below).
4. Give your money to a charity (see guidelines below).
5. Join a political party or cause committed to helping others.
6. Do a random act of kindness. A few years ago, I was walking with my sisters in the park and two of us noticed what looked like a discarded letter. We picked it up and it was a beautiful card. Inside the card were the words: 'This is a random act of kindness. Follow your bliss and have a wonderful day.' There was no name on the card. Someone had left the card there for us (or whoever else might have seen it!). I have left a few similar cards like that around and they probably made whoever read them as happy as I was when I found that one with my sisters. There is a website with a ton of ideas for random acts that do not take long: https://www.randomactsofkindness. org/kindness-ideas. You can leave sticky notes, thank-you notes, small change at a laundrette, or just smile. Use your imagination.
7. Donate something to charity. This will also help unclutter your space (most of us have way too much stuff) and make someone else happy.

Just as Sergeant Brian Grigsby and Officer Troy Dillard saved Melvyn Amrine, doing these small things will improve someone's life in a measurable way. It will probably also make you healthier. Try it and see how it feels.

A few guidelines about volunteering and doing nice things

Choose a charity with a proven track record of producing results
Many charities spend well over half the money they receive on administration, large salaries for their staff, and other costs that have nothing to do with the cause they are supposed to promote. Others promote causes that make little sense. I heard of one charity that was reportedly providing laptop computers to under-nourished children in villages with no electricity. Needless to say, laptops do not work without electricity and hungry children need food more than they need computers.

Fortunately, there are more than a few good charities. I am currently based in Oxford and the international charity based here (Oxfam) is known to be quite good, and spends over eighty per cent of the money they raise on actually relieving suffering. There are other good charities too, and to find them all you need to do is a few minutes' research on the Internet, because charities are required by law to report how they spend their money. Nobody is perfect and no organisation is perfect, but there are many that are excellent.

Give a man a fish and he'll be hungry tomorrow, teach him to fish and he'll have food for a lifetime
Focusing on long-term sustainable development will result in more lasting change. This does not mean you should force a starving person to attend your 'how to fish' class. If they need food, feed them first, then teach them how to fish. But try to help in ways that go beyond their immediate needs. There are many examples of these, and I am aware of two of them.

One is a homeless charity in Oxford called Oxford Homeless

Pathways. It gives people food and shelter, but makes sure the homeless people are connected to a health service and they have documents; it also offers courses and counselling, and even helps them to find jobs. Some of the homeless have ended up working for the shelter. Unfortunately, some of their shelters are being decommissioned over the next year.

I know of another example personally. One of the homeless people in Oxford is a guy called Hank (not his real name), who set up his bed in a bus shelter. Someone bought him some paints and he started painting and displaying his paintings on the street, which he sold. Eventually, people helped him find a government-sponsored place to stay, and he even got a job at a local restaurant where he helps out. On my birthday last year, he even got me a present of a carefully wrapped box of chocolates and a card. Simply giving him money would have helped, but not as much as helping him with the paintings, or helping him get a job. To be fair, it was easy to help Hank because he is not a substance user, he is always clean, and always polite.

Charities committed to educating women are often good for this reason, because when women are educated they can make better decisions for themselves and their families, which have a spill-over effect into their families and the societies in which they live.

Lend a helping hand
In addition to giving much-needed money, some people need to give their time. So you can offer to volunteer somewhere. Or if you are giving money, at least take a few minutes to check where the money goes.

There are lots of things you can do that can help the world and help you. The health benefits of volunteering are even greater if the reasons for volunteering are altruistic.

Takeaway 2: Show gratitude

Lots of studies show that showing gratitude plays a role in reducing depression and other anxiety disorders. Make a list of the things you had reasons to be grateful for in the last week. If you feel grateful for something someone did, express it to them.

PART V

Change Your Brain and Your DNA

Man, know thyself
        proverb of the External Temple of Luxor, Egypt

On the older view, brains and genes were perceived as unchangeable determinants of human beings. If your brain got hard-wired the wrong way when you were growing up, or you were born with the wrong genes, then it was pretty much tough luck. There was nothing you could do about it. If this were correct, there would be little point in relaxing, positive thinking, good social networks and so on, because these could not affect your genes or your brains. However, the hard evidence presented in this book calls this older view into question, and so do recent scientific experiments. Our brains and our genes may be difficult to modify, but it seems that they can change. Even our behaviour and our thoughts can affect them.

The emerging discipline of epigenetics suggests that we can have significant influence over our genes and the science of neuroplasticity suggests that you can change your brain. Because they are so sexy, epigenetics and neuroplasticity get a lot of press and a lot of promises are made on their behalf. If you believed everything you read about them, you might come away thinking it was possible to use your mind to radically transform your body and maybe even cure terminal illnesses just by thinking the right thought.

Such claims are not supported by solid evidence such as that offered by systematic reviews of randomised trials. And they might never be. There are, however, some trials showing that our environment can influence both our genes and our brains. Our genes and brains, in turn, can influence our health in a positive way. I explore this evidence in the next two chapters.

13
Nature Versus Nurture, with an Epigenetic Twist

I'm one of those people you hate because of genetics. It's the truth.

Brad Pitt

You inherit your environment just as much as your genes
Johnny Rich, American author and entrepreneur

In 2012, the actress Angelina Jolie was found to have a faulty copy of a gene called BRCA1 that her doctors claimed gave her an eighty-seven per cent chance of getting breast cancer. To prevent this, she had her breasts removed and replaced. This was supposed to reduce her risk of getting breast cancer to less than five per cent. She encouraged others to consider doing the same when she said, 'I want to encourage every woman, especially if you have a family history of breast or ovarian cancer, to seek out the information and medical experts who can help you through this aspect of your life, and to make your own informed choices.' Jolie's mother and grandmother had cancer, giving her added motivation to take action.

The question I am going to investigate in this chapter is whether her doctors were correct to say that having the BRCA1 gene gave her an eighty-seven per cent chance of getting breast cancer. It is an important question for this book, because if our health is mostly determined by our genes, what is the point of trying to do anything about it?

This is related to the age-old debate about whether our parents or our upbringing and environment are more important in shaping our traits and prospects – often called nature versus nurture. Whereas advances in genetics during the second half of the twentieth century seemed to support the power of nature, more recent discoveries in the field of epigenetics has seen the pendulum swing, giving back nurture – the environment – an equally prominent role. We will see that the environment shapes us as much as our genes, and our environment can actually affect our genetic makeup. More than that, since the cell's environment is affected by emotions and thoughts, positive thinking and relaxation can also affect our genes.

Genes as the building blocks of life

While even the earliest of cave men and women presumably would have noticed the physical similarities between children and their parents, humans only began to understand why that is the case around 150 years ago. Our bodies are made up of cells. The middle of these cells has a kind of control centre called a nucleus. Within the nucleus are things called chromosomes. The best-known chromosomes are the sex chromosomes. Females have two X chromosomes, and males have one X and one Y chromosome. There are in-between cases too, but that covers the basics. We normally get twenty-three chromosomes from our mother's egg and twenty-three from our father's sperm, and that is supposed to determine what kind of person you are.

Looking even more closely, the chromosomes are made up of large deoxyribonucleic acid (DNA) molecules. The DNA molecules contain instructions for how to build, develop and reproduce all living things and some viruses. A 'gene' is simply a section of DNA. The genes are sections that are responsible for specific parts of the body, such as eye colour, number of limbs and blood type.

The reason some believe we are largely the product of our DNA is that it carries instructions about how to make proteins. Proteins, in turn, are the building blocks of our bodies, like the bricks of a house. To name a few examples, antibodies are proteins that help protect the body against viruses, enzymes are proteins that carry out all of the chemical reactions that take place inside cells, growth hormones are proteins that help cells grow and reproduce, actin is a protein that helps muscles contract, and ferritin is a protein that stores iron and releases it in a controlled fashion.

Since humans are basically bundles of proteins built according to instructions contained in our DNA, it is no surprise that some scientists came to believe that the key to understanding our species could be found there. Accordingly, scientists set out to learn more about DNA and genes.

They found genes that determine eye colour, skin colour and height, although of course humans already knew these traits could be inherited. They also found genes that increased the risk of some diseases like haemophilia, cystic fibrosis and Huntington's disease. The hope was that the discovery of these genes would lead to the development of genetic cures for the diseases to which they were linked.

Genes were also found that seemed to influence our minds. Some studies identified gene mutations associated with autism, attention deficit hyperactivity disorder, depression, bipolar disorder and schizophrenia. It should be noted this research did not show these genetic variants *caused* these conditions, only that they were associated with them. There is even an on-going search for genes linked to happiness. All these discoveries about genes made many scientists believe that once they learned everything about genes, they would know everything about us. Forget all this positive-thinking mumbo-jumbo, they thought, let's look at genes. This line of thinking led to the launch of the Human Genome Project.

The human genome project: mega project or mega flop?

In 1990 the US Government invested $3.8 billion in the Human Genome Project. It led to some successes, including improved diagnosis of some cancers and personalised blood-thinning medication. Couples using in-vitro fertilisation can also screen their embryos for hereditary diseases. Yet the Human Genome Project and genetic medicine more broadly have not come close to revolutionising health the way that antibiotics, anaesthesia or polio vaccines did, and it has been much more costly.

The growing personalised-medicine movement that attempts to discover targeted drugs for people with certain genetic profiles has so far failed to deliver on even a fraction of the promises made for it. Cases like that of Angelina Jolie's faulty BRCA1 gene might make the headlines, but they do not really add much to what we already knew. Doctors could have told Jolie that she was at high risk of cancer, based on her family history, before the invention of the BRCA1 test. In the end, many people admit that the Human Genome Project has been an expensive flop.

In 2010, *New York Times* writer Nicholas Wade reported:

> Ten years after President Bill Clinton announced that the first draft of the human genome was complete, medicine has yet to see any large part of the promised benefits.

Worse, the human genome project revealed or confirmed several facts that undermine the very role of genes in determining what our bodies, minds and health are like.

For one, all the cells in your body, whether they are part of your hair, heart or skin, have pretty much the same DNA. Yet the cells themselves are not the same: a bone cell is very different from an eyeball cell. The DNA of bees is even weirder. Queen bees and worker bees are distinct, with the queen being large and laying eggs and the workers being small and infertile, but they have the *same* DNA. Even more puzzling is that red blood cells do not even have a nucleus or DNA, yet they still live. If the DNA is the source of our biology, how can cells and bees with the same DNA be so different?

Furthermore, scientists were surprised to learn that mice have roughly as many genes as humans (about 20,500). Even very simple species such as fruit flies and worms have about half as many genes as humans. We are more than twice as complex as worms, so why do we have only twice as many genes as worms? Even weirder is that scientists do not know what most of the genes do, with ninety-eight per cent of our DNA being classified as 'junk DNA'. If genes are that important, why are most of them junk? Stranger still, you can remove a cell's nucleus, which contains its DNA, and the cell can live for several months without changing its behaviour. Again: if DNA is the genetic blueprint that controls everything about the cell's function, how can cells survive without it?

You do not need to be a geneticist to know that a baby boy born with a gene associated with being tall will not grow up to be tall if nobody feeds him properly. And if a girl is born with a gene associated with intelligence, assuming for a moment that such a thing exists, they will not learn to understand Shakespeare if they are raised by wild animals. We all know that the environment, or nurture, plays a strong role in the development of humans and other species. The hype surrounding the Human Genome Project led to exaggerated beliefs about the importance of genes.

At the other end of the spectrum from the belief that our genes are responsible for everything is the tabula rasa, or blank slate, theory. According to this view, our environment is the only important thing and genes play no role at all.

The other extreme: the tabula rasa theory

Most contemporary psychologists believe that personalities can be modified. This should not be surprising, since if we could not modify our personalities, psychologists would all be unemployed. The American psychologist John Watson famously said if he had control of the environment a child grew up in, he could turn the infant into a doctor, lawyer, thief or a painter. Watson and fellow psychologist Burrhus Frederic Skinner believed the mind was a blank slate, or 'tabula rasa', at birth, after which we develop our traits as a result of our environments and our behaviour. They attribute everything about our personalities to nurture and none whatsoever to nature.

The 1983 comedy film *Trading Places* is about this theory. Eddie Murphy starts off as a beggar, while Dan Aykroyd is the top manager in a successful private business run by two elderly brothers. The brothers bet that they can turn Murphy into a successful manager and Aykroyd into a beggar if they change their circumstances. They take everything away from Aykroyd and give everything to Murphy and watch what happens. I won't give away the ending for those of you who haven't seen it – if not, I recommend you do purely for a good laugh.

Now if the tabula rasa theory is true, then genes do not play any role in our personalities. But just as exaggerating the role of genes is a mistake, so is downplaying the role of what we are born with. Environments can influence us, but any parent or obstetrician will tell you that their children are also born with their own personality traits. The first thing the doctor said about my sister Samantha was that she had a good set of lungs, because she cried very loudly. She doesn't scream or cry any more, yet I am sure she would be happy to acknowledge that she is still very expressive.

The same thing applies to health. Someone predisposed to cancer who decides to smoke is more likely to get cancer than someone similarly predisposed who does not smoke. In fact, common sense dictates that both nature (our genes) and nurture (our environment) play roles in both our health and our personalities. The emerging science of epigenetics even shows that the environment can influence our genes.

The mechanism and evidence for epigenetics

Jean-Baptiste Lamarck was an eighteenth-century French soldier turned biologist who believed that the environment could change a species, and what they passed on to their offspring. To Lamarck, a giraffe might develop a slightly longer neck after a lifetime of striving to reach higher and get those tasty leaves that other giraffes could not reach. Its babies would then inherit the longer neck. This ran against standard evolutionary theory, according to which a giraffe might develop a longer neck through a random genetic mutation. Then, because the giraffe with the genes for the longer neck was able to reach more leaves, they would be less likely to starve and more likely to have offspring. In this way, the accidental beneficial gene would be favoured and passed on. The outcome in Lamarck's and the standard theories is still the same: giraffes get longer necks.

However, whether humans change through random gene mutations or conscious intention has profound implications for how we approach our bodies, our relationships, and life in general. If it is all decided by our father's sperm, our mother's egg, and random genetic mutations, what is the point of striving for the human equivalent of that higher leaf? And what is the point of investing in social programmes that can help? On the other hand, if our efforts can affect our biology and even our offspring, then maybe it is worth it.

For a while, science seemed to be against Lamarck because of an experiment with mice. In 1889, German evolutionary biologist August Weismann cut off the tails of mice for twentytwo generations, and did not find that the mice tails became shorter over the generations. Against this background, American science writer Martin Gardner declared Lamarckism to be officially dead in 1957.

In fact, Gardner was wrong. Lamarck's theory was partly right, whereas Weismann's experiment was faulty. When scientists removed the mice's tails, it was not the same as when giraffes were trying to reach higher to get more leaves. Lamarck was clear that the trait passed on to further generations if it involved a wilful overcoming of obstacles. A number of studies, such as those I will discuss now, show that Lamarck was partly correct, and why this is important for our health.

Evidence for epigenetics

The more mother rats lick their pups, the less stress they have. More than that, the genes responsible for releasing stress hormones become suppressed, and this can be passed on to the next generation. Similar things can happen with humans. The rural Swedish district of Overkalix has had many famines over the last 150 years. Men whose grandfathers had endured a failed crop season, and had therefore survived starvation conditions before puberty, lived longer than men whose grandfathers had not experienced a failed crop season. In a similar study, researchers in Bristol found that men who smoked before puberty had fatter sons than those who did not. In both of these cases, changes caused by a person's environment were being passed on to offspring much later down the line.

If genes determine our biology, then there is not much we can do to affect genetic diseases (and according to genetic extremists, diseases must be genetic by definition) other than changing our genes, perhaps by doing lots of expensive research on even more expensive genetic medicine. On the other hand, if we can influence our genes, then things are, at least partly, in our hands. Professor Dean Ornish at the University of California did a trial showing the important health implications of epigenetics.

Ornish's trial involved thirty men who had a small risk of getting prostate cancer. They agreed to do yoga and exercise, switch to a low-fat diet rich in vegetables and fruits, and to take vitamin C supplements. They also agreed to go on a three-day intensive retreat. Ornish surrounded the men with the furniture, music and reading material from the time of their youth to create the same atmosphere that would have existed when they were younger. He was trying to make the men *feel* younger. After three months, the men had lower stress levels and lower cholesterol. Most significantly and surprising of all, their genes associated with the prostate cancer had changed and now indicated a lower risk. Other trials are beginning to confirm that lifestyle interventions, such as the one Ornish designed, can influence our genes.

The easiest way to understand how epigenetics works is to think of DNA as an architectural blueprint for creating proteins. The proteins, in turn, make up your body. Eric Lander, of the Massachusetts Institute of Technology, was one of the scientists who led the Human Genome Project. He explains epigenetics by analogy with a Boeing 777 aircraft. The DNA is like the parts list of the plane. You still need some instructions for how to put the parts together. The environment around the cell provides these instructions, and the instructions can be passed from generation to generation.

Even more recent than epigenetics, however, is the growing excitement around precision genome editing in the last three to four years. Might this push the pendulum in the nature–nurture debate back in the direction of nature?

Can we edit our genes like we edit a book?

Scientists in the late 1980s and early 1990s noticed something odd about the DNA of bacteria. They spotted strange repetitive sections of DNA they called 'clustered regularly interspaced short palindromic repeats' (CRISPRs). They found them to be part of a pretty cool immune-defence mechanism. Bacteria store samples of invading viruses' DNA within their own DNA between CRISPRs. They use this as an enemy mug-shot reference library that they can use to recognise and attack previously encountered viruses. Some of the key work to reveal this was published in 2007 by scientists at the Danish food company Danisco, who used the discovery to produce yoghurts and cheese that were less susceptible to viral attack.

Other scientists were quick to spot the wider potential. In 2012–13, other researchers demonstrated that the CRISPR mechanism could be used to turn off unwanted genes, or even to insert a new gene into a cell's DNA. The technique is cheaper, quicker and easier than previous genome-editing techniques, and thousands of scientists have adopted it. CRISPR has been hailed by some as among the most significant advances of the last fifty years for its ability to help scientists to target, study and therefore understand what specific parts of our DNA actually do. They also think that CRISPR might help treat or even eradicate diseases that result from genetic errors.

Whether it lives up to this potential remains to be seen. If it does and we are able to develop ways to treat or even wipe out diseases caused by genetic variants, might this show the previous optimism around genetics was justified after all? Were those who emphasised the role of nature over nurture right in the end?

In a word, no. There are some diseases that are caused by defects in single genes, as we have seen, such as cystic fibrosis and Huntingdon's Disease. The use of CRISPR to treat these and other conditions caused by single genes would be major medical breakthroughs. However, in most cases, illnesses are only partially heritable, and often environmental and lifestyle factors are more important than genes. There is also evidence that our thoughts and our minds might even be able to affect our genes.

Can our minds influence our genes?

If our genes cause happiness, sadness and depression, there is nothing we can do other than pray for the development of a therapy to fix our (un)happy genes. Epigenetics calls this into question, because it shows that even if there were a happy gene, we can probably influence it, not only for us, but for our children too. But how can we influence our genes? Many things in our environment determine which genes get expressed. They include the food you eat, the quality of the air you breathe, and whether you smoke.

Beyond bad air and food, our cells also respond to our emotional environment. Your blood is basically the immediate environment of all the cells in your body. Under stress, the body releases cortisol and adrenaline into the bloodstream. And remember that your mind is partly in control of whether you activate your stress response. So here is the cool thing: since your mind influences whether you induce the stress response, and the stress response changes the environment of your cells, and the environment of your cells determines whether certain genes are expressed, it follows that your *mind* can influence your genes.

Too much stress (often caused by not taking the time to relax and de-stress) activates the sympathetic nervous system, causing higher levels of cortisol and adrenaline in your blood. This does not just affect how you feel, it affects your DNA too. A recent systematic review including forty-three studies found that higher levels of stress hormones such as cortisol can damage your DNA by increasing the chances of unwanted gene mutations. The stress response also affects how the cells produce proteins that your body needs to grow, repair and to defend itself from diseases including cancer. All of these harmful effects are counteracted when you take the time to induce the relaxation response. When you react and act in a relaxed, loving way, cortisol and adrenaline levels do not rise to damage your DNA and your body. And, as epigenetics suggests, your offspring will be less likely to experience those negative effects of stress.

Where does this leave Angelina Jolie – and me?

The idea that our DNA determines the shape and health of our bodies, and even our personalities, left everything from our eye colour and height to our mental dispositions down to nature, our father's sperm and mother's egg. As we have just seen, the excitement surrounding the Human Genome Project reinforced the importance of genes and generated many exaggerated claims about the power of genes and therefore of genetic medicine. In a way, the science of epigenetics takes us back to common sense. Genes are important, but so is the environment. The thing epigenetics adds is that the environment does not affect us independently of our genes, environment affects the very genes we pass on to our children as well. While the field is relatively new and the extent of the influence of our environment on our genes is not fully known, it clearly shows that genes are not as important as some previously suggested.

As for Angelina Jolie, her family background made her desire to protect herself from getting breast cancer understandable and right. On top of that, cancer is a terrible, scary disease and the way people deal with it is personal. We need to respect that, and I admire Jolie's courage in making her difficult decision public.

The question here is whether having a faulty version of the BRCA1 gene gave her an eighty-seven per-cent chance of developing breast cancer as her doctors led her and then us to believe. Although I do not have access to Jolie's test results, the best evidence suggests that in most cases the chance would be closer to fifty-seven per cent. And while there are some exceptions such as the BRCA1 gene, cancer in general may be only ten per cent connected to genes.

We are going to keep reading about new genetic discoveries and medicines that will promise to unlock some secret of our biology or cure some disease. How good are these promises likely to be? In a word: not very. In most cases, illnesses are only partially heritable, and often environmental and lifestyle factors are more important than genes.

A summary of studies on twins published by Cecile Janssens, of Emory University, in Atlanta, Georgia, in 2010, estimated the genetic proportion of many diseases. Twin studies are great because identical twins have the same genes, so if they have different diseases then it must be caused by some environmental (non-genetic) factor. In the study, Janssens found that the genetic component of diseases is highly variable.

Here are a few examples of diseases and the percentage caused by genetic factors: type 2 diabetes (26 per cent), breast cancer (27 per cent), anxiety disorder (32 per cent), depression (37 per cent), prostate cancer (42 per cent), heart attack (38 per cent for men, 57 per cent for women), migraine (45 per cent), rheumatoid arthritis (53–65 per cent), obesity (75 per cent for men, 77 per cent for women), Alzheimer's disease (79 per cent), schizophrenia (81 per cent), and Type 1 diabetes (88 per cent).

Therefore, in most instances, factors like diet, exercise, air quality, stress levels and social relationships will remain important for our health and life chances no matter how far new technologies push forward the boundaries of what we know about the roles and significance of specific parts of our DNA.

Unfortunately, the exaggerated attention given to genetic factors in disease by the media means that environmental causes and preventative measures are often ignored or downplayed. This is important for understanding the science in this book, because if our genes determine our health, there is not much point in trying to think healthier thoughts or adopt better habits. On the other hand, if we know that the environment is equally important (which it is), this can motivate us to make positive changes.

Takeaway: Lifestyle interventions to reduce genetic risk factors

The lifestyle interventions such as the one in Dean Ornish's study do not only work by affecting your body and mind at the level you can see: they also affect your underlying DNA. Dean Ornish's intervention involved:

- Eating more fruit and vegetables
- Doing more exercise
- Doing yoga
- Putting yourself in a place that reminds you of your youth

Doing *all* of these things may be difficult at first; however, choosing one of them is not. Adding a large, healthy salad to your meals, and eating more fruit, takes only a tiny bit of planning. For some of us, doing exercise comes quite naturally. If it doesn't, then join an exercise group with people you like. As for putting yourself in a place that reminds you of your youth, that is very easy. Simply do something (safe and healthy) that you used to do when you were a teenager.

14
Neuroplasticity and Changing Your Brain

Be careful of your thoughts, for your thoughts become your words. Be careful of your words, for your words become your actions. Be careful of your actions, for your actions become your habits. Be careful of your habits, for your habits become your character. Be careful of your character, for your character becomes your destiny.

Chinese proverb

Insanity is doing the same thing, over and over again, but expecting different results

Albert Einstein

The hard-wired brain?

In February 1983, my grandparents were visiting my uncle and aunt in the small Canadian town of Peace River, Alberta. In the middle of the night there was a commotion and my grandfather ran upstairs from the guest room to my uncle's room and said, 'Mom is having a problem.' My uncle went down to find my grandma unable to move or speak properly. He carried her to the car, and drove her to the local hospital. She'd had a stroke in the left side of her brain. The blood and oxygen supply to that region had been cut off, leading to the death of crucial brain cells. She was in the Peace River hospital for a month before being flown to Edmonton, where she was in a rehab hospital for several weeks. Despite this, the stroke left the right side of her body paralysed.

The doctors and physiotherapists and her family focused on helping her to increase the use of the left side of her body.

Even simple tasks are difficult with only one hand. My grandma used to love squeezing fresh oranges to make juice for breakfast. However, if you think about it, you cannot do this with one hand. You need to hold the orange with one hand, while the other hand cuts. If you can't hold the orange, it tries to escape while you attempt to cut it. Before he died, my grandfather made her a cool cutting board with suction cups underneath and two nails poking up out of it. That way Grandma could stick the orange onto the nails and cut it in half with one hand, without either the cutting board or the orange trying to escape.

My maternal grandmother grew up on a ranch with no running water or much time to complain about it. Grandma was a tough lady and she lived on for another thirty years after her stroke, mostly in her own house. She changed from knitting, which requires two hands, to a kind of crocheting that requires only one. She crocheted rugs for each of her five remaining children and all eleven of her grandchildren with just her left hand. My rug is as long as me and is of a Scottish Soldier playing the bagpipes.

According to conventional medical thinking at the time of her stroke, my grandma's care and rehabilitation was a success story, because she learnt to function relatively well using only the left side of her body. Trying to get her to use her right hand would supposedly have been pointless, since the part of her long-since hard-wired brain that sends signals to the right side of the body was dead. Or so they thought.

Until recently, virtually all scientists believed that our brains become largely fixed during what are called sensitive or critical periods in childhood, at a time when brain circuits are unusually open to being shaped by sensory experiences. According to this view, each part of the brain is responsible for a specific function in the body. For example, the visual cortex (located at the back of the brain) is responsible for visual perception, the auditory cortex (located to the side of the brain just above the ears) is responsible for making sense of sounds, and the motor cortex (in the top, middle of the brain) is responsible for moving limbs, and so on.

Knowing which parts of the brain were responsible for specific functions allowed scientists to create a 'brain map'. The development of technology for brain imaging such as computed axial tomography (CAT), magnetic resonance imaging (MRI), and functional magnetic resonance imaging (fMRI) seemed to support the view that brains were hard-wired. Brain imaging showed that different parts of our brains were responsible for moving our hands, for vision and for interpreting sounds. Since the brain was seen as hard-wired, nothing could be done about the paralysis of the right side of the body in someone who had suffered a stroke in the left side of their brain, like my grandmother. Story over then?

In fact, as is often the case in science, a story that seemed over was not. Medical conventional wisdom on the degree to which the brain can be rewired in adulthood has changed. Had my grandma had her stroke ten years later, the chances are that she would have regained control of her right arm.

Paul Bach-Y-Rita and his father

In 1958, University of Wisconsin Professor Paul Bach-Y-Rita's father Pedro suffered a stroke. Like in my grandmother's case, half of his body was paralysed. He also lost his ability to speak. Paul's psychiatrist brother, George, refused to believe that Pedro would spend the rest of his days in this condition and dedicated his life to helping him. George kept encouraging Pedro to try and use the paralysed side of his body, and eventually – after a lot of hard work – he did. Pedro got to the point where he could walk and hike normally. An autopsy performed on Pedro's body when he died revealed that he had suffered serious damage to his brain stem, which had not repaired itself after the stroke. While areas of the brain damaged by the stroke had remained so until Pedro died, other parts seemed to have taken over control of the paralysed side of the body to allow it to move again.

His father's recovery inspired Paul Bach-Y-Rita to conduct a daring and fascinating experiment in which he tried to teach blind people to see with their tongues. Most blind people's eyes work, it is the connection between the eyes and the brain that does not. You don't just see with your eyes, you see with your mind and brain. The eye sends signals to a part of your brain near the back of your skull called the visual cortex. Your consciousness then perceives those signals to tell you what the thing is in the visual cortex. The same goes for what you hear, and feel, and smell.

When most people go blind, what they really lose is the ability to transmit signals from the eye via the optic nerve to the visual cortex. Noting this, Bach-Y-Rita sought to teach the brain how to see via the sensation of touch. In one example, he developed a device that translated images on a camera placed on the heads of blind people into patterns of sensations delivered to their tongues by a special ribbon. For instance, if the camera saw something square, it would cause sensations in the shape of a square to be delivered to the tongue. The blind person would then feel something shaped like a square on their tongue and know that there was a square-shaped thing in front of them. They increased the complexity of the things people 'saw' until eventually several patients were able to recognise the supermodel Twiggy. The study was all the more dramatic because the blind people in the experiments were congenitally blind, meaning they had never been able to see.

These experiments sparked a new field called sensory substitution that is currently a hot topic leading to many potentially important clinical applications. The experiments also led to the foundation of the science of neuroplasticity. The word neuroplasticity comes from the root words Neuron and Plastic. A neuron is a nerve cell in the brain, and plastic is used in the sense of to mould, sculpt or modify.

Neuroplasticity refers to the potential that the brain has to reorganise itself by creating new neural pathways. While Bach-Y-Rita's experiments all happened years before my grandma had her stroke, the results were not implemented into mainstream stroke rehabilitation. This was partly because science can move at a frustratingly slow pace, and also because the view that the brain was hard-wired was difficult to overthrow. This all changed when animal experiments provided some insight into the underlying mechanisms explaining how the brain changes.

Discovery of how the brain can change

In the late 1970s and early 1980s, neuroscientist Professor Edward Taub conducted some experiments on monkeys in Silver Spring, Maryland, that explained what happened when the brain was being rewired. He started by cutting the monkeys' nerves that sent signals from one of their limbs to the brain. For example, he would cut the nerves that communicated between a monkey's right arm and brain, so it could not move the arm. He then restricted the left arm, forcing the monkey to try and use the 'bad' right arm. Eventually these animals would relearn to use their bad limbs, meaning they had been reconnected to the nervous system.

Soon after his initial experiments, Edward Taub was charged with animal cruelty and he had to stop his experiments. Animal rights activists argued that the animals were not treated humanely. After a long and hard-fought battle, all the charges against Taub were eventually dropped as being baseless. But the protestors had a point: Bach-Y-Rita proved that we could have learned the same thing without inflicting what to many people was cruelty towards the monkeys. Experiments such as those carried out by Taub could not only have avoided legal and ethical issues, but also concerns about whether the results of research on monkeys apply to humans.

Taub's work was eventually adapted for use with humans

who had suffered from strokes in a kind of treatment called Constraint Induced Movement Therapy. This involves placing the limb that can be used in a sling, splint, or restricting its movement in some other way, for ninety per cent of the patient's waking hours for about two weeks. The therapy has been shown to be highly effective for people who have suffered a stroke. Had the therapy been common when my grand-mother first had her stroke, I have no doubt that with her determined character she would have completely recovered most of the use of her right side.

The science of neuroplasticity and how the brain changes is flourishing, and experiments have even shown that the brain can generate new neurons, and that this can happen in elderly people. It can also happen faster than was previously believed. Researchers who carried out scans on medical students before and after they studied for exams found the volume of grey matter in their brains increased significantly in a matter of months.

How your brain can change

Change can help us survive, so from an evolutionary perspec-tive it is hardly surprising that our brains can be remoulded. Humans are considered to be the most adaptable species on the planet. Even rats and cockroaches cannot live in places like Iceland, where humans have thrived for centuries. This ability to learn to survive in climates ranging from scorching hot deserts to freezing cold northern tundra has been a major evolutionary advantage. If our ancestors' brains were hard-wired, humans could not have learned to adapt and thrive in the climates we now inhabit.

You may recall from earlier chapters that our physiological responses to the world around us are not only caused by external stimuli, but also by the way we interpret and react to them. The way we react, in turn, is determined partly by our neural networks. Let's say two people in a room see a spider on the window. One of them is frightened of spiders and experiences a fight-or-flight response. To the other, the sight reminds them of a cuddly spider toy they had as a child and it gives them a warm, nostalgic feeling. News of rain might upset someone planning a picnic, while bringing a smile to the face of a farmer whose crops need water. A paranoid person night think that someone looking at them is planning to rob them, whereas a more confident person might perceive the same lingering look as a sign that the same person is attracted to them.

Key differences in these examples are in the ways the brains of the different individuals have learned to react. How does the perception of a spider activate the fight-or-flight response in one person or the warm nostalgic response of another? Here is what is going on within the brain. The visual cortex communicates with the amygdala, which is responsible for activating the fight-or-flight response, via nervous system cells called neurons.

Neurons rarely connect randomly with other neurons. Instead, they connect via neural networks that are a bit like groups of well-worn roads. As soon as a person who is scared of spiders sees the object of their fear, the brain network that links the image to the amygdala activates. For the person who grew up with a stuffed, friendly spider toy, the perception of a spider is strongly connected to parts of the brain that generate feel-good chemicals.

The creation of neural networks based on experience is what allows us to learn. When a child puts their finger close to a flame they feel pain. This creates a neural network connecting the perception of fire and parts of the brain that warns us to stay away. This helps us to avoid getting burned. Next time you are near a candle, try to put your fingers near the flame. You can almost feel the signal in your brain applying the brakes to your hand. You do not need to consciously think about avoiding a flame, it all happens naturally.

Other habits include looking both ways before you cross

the road, driving or walking a familiar route, for example from home to work, reaching in your pocket to get a wallet when you are paying for something, and indeed most of the things we do every day. These subconscious learnt habits are useful because they free our minds up to do other more productive things. If we had to constantly remember or relearn that flames burn, that our money is in our wallets, or that there are dangerous cars on the streets, we would have little energy left to do much else. That these neural network-based behaviours are automatic is usually useful, but they are also a double-edged sword, as we can develop patterns that are bad for us.

Eating chocolate cake gives us a dopamine high, which in turn teaches our brains that doing so makes us feel good. This is fine up to a point; however, it can lead to two problems. First, too much chocolate cake can be bad for our health and, second, it can make us falsely generalise from one emotional experience. Someone who has been hurt in a relationship might come to think that getting close to people generally leads to getting hurt, in the same way that we might react to putting our hands close to flames. The same thing can apply to sex, drugs and emotional reactions to things. For example, someone who gets their own way by shouting as a child may become angry as their default reaction when people disagree with them. Neuroplasticity offers us an escape from these patterns.

What neuroplasticity means for you: changing habits

Most of us now live in an era in which cardiovascular diseases (CVD), such as heart attacks and strokes, are more likely to kill us than infectious illnesses like tuberculosis and pneumonia that killed our ancestors. Unlike infectious diseases, cardiovascular diseases are more successfully treated by lifestyle changes to our eating and exercise habits than medicine. Even the risk of cancer can be greatly reduced by maintaining a healthy lifestyle. The bad news is that eating less and exercising more is easier said than done. The good news is that besides helping people recover from strokes, neuroplasticity suggests that it really is possible to change our brains and our habits. Let's look at habits in a bit more detail.

Habits are automatic behaviours triggered by cues that produce a reward. Pulling your hand away from a flame to avoid getting burned is automatic. The flame is the cue to pull your hand away (behaviour) to get a reward (avoid getting burned). An urge to sneeze is a cue to cover your mouth with your hand to avoid people telling you off – depending, of course, on your upbringing. So the pattern is: cue → behaviour → reward.

In his book about changing habits, the American writer Charles Duhigg talks about how he changed his habit of eating a chocolate cookie every afternoon. His cue was that he became bored in the middle of the afternoon, so he developed a habit of walking to the cafeteria to speak with his friends. In the cafeteria, his routine was to buy a chocolate cookie. His reward was feeling refreshed because he'd had a break from work. From a neuroscientific point of view, Duhigg trained his brain to get up from his desk, walk to the cafeteria, buy a cookie, and then feel rewarded and ready for more work in the afternoon. The sense of satisfaction he got as a result was in fact a dopamine rush that he came to crave, leading him to continue performing his afternoon cookie ritual.

To change his habit, Duhigg had to interrupt the cue → behaviour → reward cycle in a new way that gave him a similar reward but without the chocolate cookie. This he did by going for a walk to get a breath of fresh air when he felt the cue (feeling bored in the afternoon). This made him feel good too, and did not involve chocolate. Until he formed a new habit, he would not have been able to go to the cafeteria and chat with his friends for a break without a cookie and still feel good about it. This is because the cafeteria provided the context which automatically triggered the cookie-buying behaviour.

One problem with habits is that they are very like addictions. An important difference is that with an addiction you need more and more to get the same rush. Try to recall the buzz you got the first time you tried coffee or alcohol. A single cup or glass was probably enough to produce an effect. Then, if you carried on drinking coffee or alcohol on a daily basis, you needed more to feel the way you did that first time. You may or may not remember, but there was a time when we were all cheap dates. The neurological explanation for this is that the neural network linking the stimulus with the reward becomes strengthened and reinforced with repeated exposures. Your body becomes accustomed to the chemicals generated by drinking coffee and beer, meaning it needs more and more in order to get excited about it.

In spite of the distinction, the difference between a habit and an addiction is a matter of degree. Addictions involve more intense cravings and usually have more detrimental effects.They both involve an automatic cue → behaviour → reward process. It is a thought pattern with its foundations within a neural network. More generally, the ways we react to things are also often habitual. They could be seen as emotional habits or addictions.

Someone who is easily angered will have a well-used neural network that activates the anger emotion. Compared to other people, signals travel easily along the network, meaning it does not take much to make the person angry. And just as someone who takes cocaine regularly will desensitise the reward pathways, the person who gets angry easily needs less and less provocation to become angry, or has to react more and more forcefully to feel the same emotion.

The same thing applies to other emotions like depression, sadness and attraction. It explains why sex addicts often need harder- and harder-core pornography to satisfy their desires.

These emotions are generated by neural networks that give your brain the associated chemical that it is used to. To change our habits we need to reprogramme the cue → behaviour → reward cycle in ways that benefit us.

Neuroplasticity provides the basis for improving habits (but doesn't give you the will to change)

Understanding that the brain is not totally hard-wired can play the same motivational role as understanding that your health is not (just) due to your genes. You really can change.

This does not mean that changing habits is easy. It is not. At a deeper level, accessing your inner will or desire to change can be difficult too. Someone might understand the science of neuroplasticity, and they might know that if they changed their thoughts about food they could eat more healthily and lose weight. But the problem many people have is that they don't have the will power. They know that healthy food is better for their bodies at an intellectual level, but they do not know how to translate that into new habits.

It is a problem I can empathise with. Whereas I am very disciplined about getting enough exercise, I love sweet things, especially Nutella. If there is any Nutella in the house and there is also a spoon, the chances are that I will eat the entire jar by the end of the day. I am well aware this is not good for me, but I find it difficult to resist, as I have had a sweet tooth since I can remember. Where can we get the will power to change these difficult things? An important part of the answer to this question is simple: believe that you can change. The mere belief that you can change will give you a dopamine rush that makes you feel good, and this can help you change your habit. This was illustrated in the discussion of self efficacy in Chapter Eight. And if you cannot muster a real belief that you can do it, start by pretending that you can. Fake it until you make it. The good thing is that if you are reading this book, you have already proven that you have some motivation.

Takeaway: Change an old habit and create a new one

Changing an old habit

Think of a habit you would like to change, and write down what the cue, behaviour and reward is. Duhigg's cue was feeling bored, his behaviour was buying a cookie, and his reward was basically a sugar high. I have the same type of habit as Duhigg and I eat too many sweet things. My cue is that I will see a sweet thing (cue), eat it (behaviour), and get a reward (a sugar high). So the next time I walk past a sweet thing, I am going to take ten deep breaths and stretch.

Creating a new habit

I'm not aware of any trials that support this exercise but it has helped me get 'unstuck' at times. Sometimes the best way to change an old habit can be to ignore it for a while and focus on something new. To create new habits and new neural pathways you have to behave in a new way. The exercise in this chapter is very simple: just do something different. Anything. It can be a big thing or a small thing. Here are some examples for inspiration:

- Eat pizza for breakfast.
- Smile and say hello to a random person on the street.
- Do something that embarrasses you.
- Try going a whole day pretending that your left hand is dominant (if your right hand is usually dominant, otherwise use your right hand): brush your teeth, eat your cereal, and write with just your left hand.
- Wear a suit and tie to work, if you don't usually do so.
- Wear jeans and a colourful T-shirt to work if you normally wear a suit and tie, unless this will cause you to lose your job, of course.
- Give your mother-in-law (or someone else you normally

don't get along with) a random telephone call and tell her you were thinking of her.

It has to be something you would not normally do. Notice how you feel when you think of it. Chances are you might feel some resistance, some reason not to do it. And when you actually do it, chances are you will feel good. Use this as a starting point to kick an old habit and start a new one.

15
Conclusion

What This All Means for You and Your Health

Man, know thyself, and you are going to know the gods
proverb of the Inner Temple of Luxor, Egypt

*If I had asked people what they wanted, they would have
said faster horses*

Henry Ford

The first year I tried to row for the Canadian rowing team, I was training like a demon twice or three times per day. I remember being so tired at night that I was barely strong enough to lift the fork to eat my dinner. Whatever I was doing was not enough, because I failed to pass the final test, and was cut from the team. I was completely devastated. After a few days of feeling depressed, I realised I was not ready to give up. The problem was that I really felt as if I was at my physical limit. What more could I do?

As I mentioned in Chapter Six, I often felt so nervous before the races that I was drained for the races themselves. I was short for an international rower and the need to outperform taller, stronger athletes meant that I could not afford to waste any energy. It was then that I remembered stories I had read about mothers lifting cars to save their children, and Yogis in India not eating for days, or standing on one leg for weeks. If I could learn to focus my mind like that, I thought, I will be able to row faster. My rational mind told me that these stories of extreme human performance through deep mental focus were probably nonsense, but I was willing to try if they would help me win. I decided to seek out a yoga teacher.

The problem was that I did not know anyone who taught traditional yoga. These people, I thought, were what I needed to control my mind and help me do the rowing equivalent of lifting cars. Yoga was not as popular back then in the mid-1990s as it is today. The few teachers I did know focused on physical postures and stretching rather than on mind over matter. Eventually, my mother (who was into that kind of stuff) put me in touch with a traditional yoga instructor in Montreal called Dr Madan Bali, whom I mentioned briefly in the Preface.

I was intrigued when I heard he had worked with the Montreal Canadiens professional ice-hockey team a few years earlier, at a time when they used to be the best team in the league. We spoke briefly on the phone and set up an appointment to meet the next day. When I got to his place, my first reaction was surprise at its modesty. The small living-room of his apartment in downtown Montreal doubled as his yoga studio. I remember the smell of curry being cooked in the kitchen, which was only separated from the living-room studio by a thin, beaded curtain. He clearly was not in it for the money.

We sat down together and I fired a battery of sceptical questions at Dr Bali. How do you know it works? If it is so great, why doesn't everyone do it? Is it scientific? What do you mean we only use two per cent of our brains? Can we really rewire our brains and our DNA? Where did you get your PhD? Dr Bali answered all my questions patiently, and his friendly manner disarmed me. It was hard to continue my aggressive line of questioning when he was being so kind, patient and informative. He told me about endorphins, about the body's ability to change, about the damage caused by the fight-or-flight response, and the power of the mind over the body.

Eventually I ran out of questions, and although I did not believe it, I wanted to believe what Dr Bali said about the mind controlling the body. If I could control my mind, I could improve my rowing performance. I was silent as I thought about these things. He smiled and told me that the first class was free so I could try it, and test for myself whether my mind felt calmer or not. I was still very suspicious, and I even wondered whether he was planning to hypnotise me and turn me into a cult member. But the offer of a free class, combined with my desperation to win races, won out against my scepticism. I decided to give it a go.

It turned out to be one of the best decisions I have ever made. Dr Bali blew me away. He was already seventy years old and could do as many leg-lifts and push-ups as I could and I was in world-class shape. More than that, I was so relaxed at the end of the session that I almost fell asleep. When I sat up, everything seemed clear. I felt deeply focused. If I could learn to control when I felt relaxed and to focus so well, I thought, I will save energy and win more races. So that is just what I did. I learned his routine, and practised yoga. Eight months after that first yoga session, I made the Canadian rowing team. But I'm not telling this story because of me, I am telling it because of Dr Bali.

Now at ninety-three years young, Dr Bali's schedule includes teaching about forty hours per week, travelling to faraway places like Indonesia to give yoga courses, and taking care of his family. He always has a smile on his face. He took care of his wife who was very ill until she passed away in 2016. His many students plague him with their trials and tribulations on a daily basis and he listens carefully and offers them good advice. I am sure he has physical and emotional aches and pains; however, he chooses to be positive and not let these things get in the way. This lets him get on with his life. That means doing exercise and interacting with people, which benefit his health. This, in turn, allows him to continue exercising and interacting. It is a virtuous circle. He says his daily practice of yoga keeps him young and healthy.

A sceptic might say that Dr Bali was born with good genes,

and that is why he is so healthy and happy at ninety-three years young. To them, his state has nothing to do with yoga. It is true that Dr Bali was born with great genes. I know this because of what he told me about a faded tattoo he has on his arm. I asked him what it was and he said it was his name, 'M. Bali'. I asked him why he had it. He replied that as a Hindu during the 1947 partition of India he had survived multiple attempts on his life as he escaped to Delhi. He thought he might not survive and wanted to make sure that anyone who found his body would recognise him so he could have a proper burial. He survived hard times that might have killed a weaker person.

So Dr Bali is not absolute *proof* that his lifestyle and attitude are what keep him going. That would require an impossible randomised trial in which his health outcomes were measured against those of a cloned version of him engaging in some tricky-to-design placebo version of traditional yoga. Such a trial would be impossible, yet at the same time, you would be hard pressed to find someone working full time and taking care of people at ninety-three years young who is not doing yoga or something similar. His story – together with the science presented in this book – suggests quite clearly that genes are not the whole picture. Dr Bali's lifestyle choices must play an important role in his health and vitality.

In a way, this book is a scientific answer to the barrage of questions I fired at Dr Bali when I first met him. My studies, and other studies, show that relaxation reduces stress and improves health, positive thinking activates the body's inner pharmacy to reduce pain, depression and anxiety, good social networks make you live longer, the care of an empathetic doctor can be just as effective as a blockbuster drug. These things might even be able to change your genes and your brain. Beyond that, the health of the different parts of your body are connected, the health of your mind and body can't be separated, and your overall health is linked to the people who surround you. The high-quality evidence presented here means that this can no longer be viewed as fuzzy, feel-good stuff: it is hard science.

I like it, but you don't need to be into yoga or meditation to benefit from what I've written. I've provided more 'neutral' exercise options that can be equally beneficial. By engaging with the exercises I hope that you have become the main character of the book and experienced the science of self-healing for yourself. I hope you now know you're not a mindless machine damned to sit back and pray for pills to cure you of the many common ills for which you currently seek medical attention.

Epilogue

What if something really serious happens?

When talking about this book, people often ask:

'This placebo stuff might help some things. But what if you had something really serious? For example what if a doctor said you needed heart surgery. Would you take a placebo or would you have the operation?'

Dan Moerman (who I quoted in this book) inspired how I think about these things. If a doctor told me I needed heart surgery, the first thing I would do is get a second opinion. We need a second opinion before agreeing to any serious or dangerous procedure. If there were another less invasive option (the way I had the option of physiotherapy and yoga for my back and knee problems) I'd start with that. But if the second opinion were the same as the first, I would probably go ahead with the operation. I would try to get an experienced surgeon with a good track record who made me feel confident and cared for. A surgeon like Bruce Moseley. I would insist that he or she do the least invasive procedure possible. I would try to get a nice room with a good view, and to have occupational therapists take care of me afterwards. I would ask all my close friends and family members to visit before, during, and after.

If I needed painkillers after the operation, I would take them the same way I take any pill on the rare occasions when I need them. On these unusual occasions, I put the pills in my hand, and say, 'You are the best, the most powerful, and trouble-free drugs in the world.' Then, with a carefully poured glass of water ('Water is good for me too,' I would say to myself), I swallow the pills, and anticipate a speedy recovery.

A friend once watched me do this and asked, 'How sure are you that these pills are helping?'

I replied, 'I'm positive.'

Acknowledgements

This book was a lot of fun to write, and I learned a great deal along the way. It also took up most of my free evenings for more than two years. I could not have done it without the help of many people. There were so many that I will undoubtedly have left some out – if you find your name is missing, get in touch and I will buy you a cup of tea and give you a free copy of the book.

I have become more grateful for my family than ever before. Especially my sister Samantha, who supported me to keep going and gave me the idea for the cover. My other sisters Katie and Teresa encouraged me, and my father gave me good advice. My cousins John and Brett gave me good ideas and solid friendship, and my cousin George went out of his way to give me some brilliant ideas. Claire was very supportive. I have got a large, extended family and I cannot name them all here: you are all special to me.

My friends, Bent, PK, Colin, Cynthia, David, Devika, Dennis, Foad, Heather, Mark, Isabel, Jurgita, Monika, Marcus, Martin, Eloïse, Jason, Renaud and Sam, were all there for me. Qarim is more creative than I will ever be and he encouraged me to think visually about the message for the cover and website. Sebastien has been my best friend since I was two years old and he has done more favours for me than I can count; I am in his debt. He gave me a ton of advice about the legal aspects of publishing. I have not rowed much with the Molesey Leg-Ends, but their daily updates keep me inspired, and the Headington Roadrunners provided a welcome distraction. John Webster is a great teacher. Inevitably I spent a lot of time in cafés and the staff at Branca were great.

Father Gavriil kind of adopted me as his spiritual son and tried to keep me on the right track. My former rowing coaches Scott Armstrong and Dusan Kovacevic are an on-going source of sound guidance about my work and life in general. The Venerable Dr Khammai Dhammasami, and Dr Pannyawamsa of Oxford Buddhist Vihara, let me stay at their monastery for a few days to complete the manuscript: it is amazing how much you can get done without any distractions.

My colleagues Jeffrey Aronson, Nancy Cartwright, Alexander Bird, Sir Muir Gray, Sir Iain Chalmers, Donald Gillies, George Lewith, Ted Kaptchuk, Mike Kelly, Frank Miller, Dan Moerman and Paul Glasziou are very different, but share a commitment to high-quality research that attempts to make things better. They hold up a high standard that I strive for and rarely achieve. I did a lot of the scientific research reported here while working with Paul Aveyard and the Behavioural Medicine Group at Oxford. The group is more supportive than any group I've ever worked with. Karin read the chapters on epigenetics and Steph helped with the conclusion. Mingy is the herbal doctor I talked about in the Preface. Donna Lee encouraged me to believe in my writing.

The book would not have seen the light of day without a publisher. I am grateful to Rupert Sheldrake for introducing me to Mark Booth at Hodder & Stoughton. It has been a real pleasure working with Mark, he is everything one could hope for in a publisher and more. Fiona the editor and Barry the copy editor were also a great help. My agent Robert Lecker helped with the formalities, and Lawrence helped kick it all off. Nic Fleming did some final editing, helped me with the CRISPR science, and generally helped make my mediocre writing a bit less mediocre.

Two people deserve a special mention. Jo Marchant interviewed me for her wonderful book *Cure*, even though she knew I was writing a book on a related topic. While our books are complementary, a less magnanimous person might have seen them as competition. Far from viewing me as a threat, she invited me to join her for a public talk at the Wellcome Trust, and made a special mention of my book at her own book launch. Her generous spirit is something I strive to emulate. Finally, my yoga teacher Dr Madan Bali is ninety-three years young and has been an ongoing source of inspiration.

Works Cited

Preface

Your body makes its own morphine (endorphins)

Stefano, G. B., et al. (2012), 'Endogenous morphine: up-to-date review 2011', Folia Biol (Praha), 58 (2), 49–56.

Side effects of antidepressants

Lilly USA LLC (2009). Medication Guide (PROZAC).

National Institutes of Health. (2017). Antidepressant Medications for Children and Adolescents: Information for Parents and Caregivers. Retrieved from https://http://www.nimh.nih.gov/health/topics/child-and-adolescent-mental-health/antidepressant-medications-for-children-and-adolescents-information-for-parents-and-caregivers.shtml.

Arroll, B., et al. (2005), 'Efficacy and tolerability of tricyclic antidepressants and SSRIs compared with placebo for treatment of depression in primary care: a meta-analysis', Ann Fam Med, 3 (5), 449–56.

Saperia, J., Ashby, D., and Gunnell, D. (2006), 'Suicidal behaviour and SSRIs: updated meta-analysis', BMJ, 332 (7555), 1453.

Placebo knee surgery as good as real knee surgery

Buchbinder, R., et al. (2009), 'A randomized trial of vertebroplasty for painful osteoporotic vertebral fractures', N Engl J Med, 361 (6), 557–68.

Introduction

The amazing advances of modern medicine

LeFanu, James (2000), The Rise and Fall of Modern Medicine (London: Abacus).

One in 7 boys in the US are diagnosed with ADHD and most of them medicated with metamphetamines

Bloom, B. and Cohen, R.A. (2007), 'Summary health statistics for U.S. Children: national health interview survey, 2007', in National Center for Health Statistics and Vital Health Statistics, (10; Washington DC).

Evidence that one in 10 adults are on antidepressants

Andrade, L., et al. (2003), 'The epidemiology of major depressive episodes: results from the international consortium of psychiatric epidemiology (ICPE) surveys', *Int J Methods Psychiatr Res*, 12 (1), 3–21.

Claim that everyone over 50 should be put on statins

Mittal, M. and Fay, W. P. (2013), 'Almost everyone over 50 should be put on a statin to reduce the risk of cardiovascular disease: a contrarian view', *Mo Med*, 110 (4), 339–41.

Elderly population take too many pills

Canada Institute for Health Information (2014), 'Drug use among seniors on public drug programs in Canada, 2012' (Ottawa, Canada: Canada Institute for Health Information).

Duerden, M., Avery, T., and Payne, R. (2013), 'Polypharmacy and medicines optimisation. Making it safe and sound' (London: The King's Fund).

Rambhade, S., et al. (2012), 'A survey on polypharmacy and use of inappropriate medications', *Toxicol In*, 19 (1), 68–73.

The prevalence of polypharmacy (taking too many pills): the harms it causes

Maher, R. L., Hanlon, J., and Hajjar, E. R. (2014), 'Clinical consequences of polypharmacy in elderly', *Expert Opin Drug Saf*, 13 (1), 57–65.

Golchin, N., et al. (2015), 'Polypharmacy in the elderly', *J Res Pharm Pract*, 4 (2), 85–8.

Trumic, E., et al. (2012), 'Prevalence of polypharmacy and drug interaction among hospitalized patients: opportunities and responsibilities in pharmaceutical care', *Mater Sociome*, 24 (2), 68–72.

Evidence that antipsychotic drugs are given to healthy older people to prevent possible psychosis

Bruser, D. and McLean, J. (2014), 'Use of antipsychotics soaring at Ontario nursing homes', *The Toronto Star*, 15 April.

Hirota, T. and Kishi, T. (2013), 'Prophylactic antipsychotic use for postoperative delirium: a systematic review and meta-analysis', *J Clin Psychiatry*, 74 (12), e1136–44.

Trials showing that 'deprescribing' (taking away medications from people who are taking many drugs) usually makes them live longer
Page, A. T., et al. (2016), 'The feasibility and the effect of deprescribing in older adults on mortality and health: a systematic review', *Br J Clin Pharmacol*.

Evidence that more people die from prescription painkillers than cocaine and heroin
Centers for Disease Control and Prevention (2015), 'Policy impact: prescription painkiller overdoses', http://www.cdc.gov/homeand recreationalsafety/rxbrief/%3E, accessed 20 January.

Evidence that medical error is the third leading cause of death in the US
Makary, M. A. and Daniel, M. (2016), 'Medical error – the third leading cause of death in the US', BMJ, 353, i2139.

Side effects of prescription drugs kill over 100,000 people in the US each year
Lazarou, J., Pomeranz, B. H., and Corey, P. N. (1998), 'Incidence of adverse drug reactions in hospitalized patients: a meta-analysis of prospective studies', *JAMA*, 279 (15), 1200–5.

Cost of prescription drugs in the US
Constantino, T. (2015), 'IMS health forecasts global drug spending to increase 30 per cent by 2020, to $1.4 trillion, as medicine use gap narrows' (Quintiles IMS).

Cost of prescription drug spending in Canada
Canadian Institute for Health Information (2015), 'Canadians spent $28.8 billion on prescription drugs in 2014' (Canadian Institute for Health Information).

Cost of healthcare spending in UK
ukpublicspending.co.uk. Public spending details for 2006. 2016. http://www.ukpublicspending.co.uk/year_spending_2006UK bn_15bc1n_10 - ukgs302.

Claim that all (or at least most) modern medicine is bad can be found here

Mercola, J. (2016), 'The Terrifying Side Effects of Prescription Drugs', <http://articles.mercola.com/sites/articles/archive/2008/04/12/the-terrifying-side-effects-of-prescription-drugs.aspx%3E, accessed 25 November.

Evidence that 80 per cent of US patient groups are funded by industry in order to promote so-called 'diseases' that aren't what many would consider to be diseases

McCarthy, M. (2017), 'More than 80% of US patients' groups take industry funds, study finds', *BMJ*, *356*, j1180. doi: 10.1136/bmj.j1180.

Description of, and examples of, 'disease mongering'

Moynihan, R., Heath, I., and Henry, D. (2002), 'Selling sickness: the pharmaceutical industry and disease mongering', *BMJ*, 324(7342), 886–891.

Claim that alternative medicine is all nonsense

The Original Sceptical Raptor (2016), 'Pseudoscience and science – alternative medicine is bullshit', http://www.skepticalraptor.com/skepticalraptorblog.php/pseudoscience-and-science-alternative-medicine-is-bullshit/%3E, accessed 25 November.

Explanation of the 'tools' of modern medicine (randomised trials and systematic reviews)

Evans, I., Thornton, H., and Chalmers, I. (2010), *Testing Treatments: Better Research forBetter Healthcare* (London: Pinter & Martin).

Evidence of the problem with unpublished trials

This website contains a database of systematic reviews showing that half of trials are unpublished: http://www.alltrials.net/news/half-of-all-trials-unreported/.

(Evidence for the health benefits of positive thinking, empathetic doctors, social networks, and how these might influence your brain and DNA are in their own chapters in the book.)

Part I

Ha-Joon Chang quote. Ha-Joon's book is also similar in that it is both 'much less and much more' than (in his case) a standard economics textbook and (in my case) a standard self-help book.

Chang, H-J. (2010) 23 *Things They Don't Tell You About Capitalism* (London: Allen Lane).

Book that traces the successes of modern medicine (ironically, the author says they arise due to chance)

LeFanu, James (2000), *The Rise and Fall of Modern Medicine* (London: Abacus).

Chapter 1

Quote about a cold going away in a week

Patulin Clinical Trials Committee, Medical Research Council (2004), 'Clinical trial of patulin in the common cold. 1944', *Int J Epidemiol*, 33 (2), 243–6.

Archie Cochrane's story about the prisoner of war camp

Cochrane, A. L. and Blythe, M. (1989), *One Man's Medicine: An Autobiography of Professor Archie Cochrane* (London: BMJ).

Life expectancy tables

Roser, M., (2016), 'Life expectancy'. Published online at OurWorldInData.org. Retrieved from: http://ourworldindata.org/data/population-growth-vital-statistics/life-expectancy/ [Online Resource]

Number of cells in human body

Sender, R., Fuchs, S., and Milo, R. (2016), 'Revised estimates for the number of human and bacteria cells in the body', *PLOS Biol*, 14 (8), e1002533.

Description of selection bias, where certain people (in the case of Cochrane's story, young healthy people) are selected for a study or group

Howick, J. (2011), *The Philosophy of Evidence-Based Medicine* (Oxford: Wiley-Blackwell).

Reference to fact that your bones are stronger than steel

University of Cambridge (2015), 'Mechanical properties of bone', http://www.doitpoms.ac.uk/tlplib/bones/bone_mechanical.php

Reference to fact that your stomach acid can melt steel

Li, P. K., et al. (1997), 'In vitro effects of simulated gastric juice on swallowed metal objects: implications for practical management', *Gastrointest Endosc*, 46 (2), 152–5.

Reference to fact that you have between 10 and 100 trillion cells in your body

Bianconi, E., et al. (2013), 'An estimation of the number of cells in the human body', *Ann Hum Biol*, 40 (6), 463–71.

Reference about number of neurons and neural connections in the human brain

Azevedo, F. A., et al. (2009), 'Equal numbers of neuronal and non-neuronal cells make the human brain an isometrically scaled-up primate brain', *J Comp Neurol*, 513 (5), 532–41.

Reference to fact that your skin regenerates itself in less than a month

American Academy of Dermatology (2015), 'How skin grows', http://www.aad.org/dermatology-a-to-z/for-kids/about-skin/how-skin-grows%3E, accessed 9 May.

General anatomy and physiology

Tortora, G.J., Derrickson, B., and Prezbindowski, K., Schmidt Learning Guide (2006), *Principles of Anatomy and Physiology, Learning Guide* (11th edn; Hoboken, NJ: John Wiley & Sons).

Cell age in human body

Spalding, K. L., et al. (2005), 'Retrospective birth dating of cells in humans', *Cell*, 122 (1), 133–43.

General immune system
Parham, P. (2009), *The Immune System* (3rd edn; London: Garland Science).

Nerve signals travel almost 300 kilometres per hour
Cummins, K. L. and Dorfman, L. J. (1981), 'Nerve fiber conduction velocity distributions: studies of normal and diabetic human nerves', *Ann Neurol*, 9 (1), 67–74.

How natural killer cells work
Topham, N. J. and Hewitt, E. W. (2009), 'Natural killer cell cytotoxicity: how do they pull the trigger?', *Immunology*, 128 (1), 7–15.

Your liver can almost completely regenerate itself
Bird, T. and Iredale, J. (2011), 'Liver regeneration by hepatic progenitor cells', Thesis (Ph.D.) (University of Edinburgh).

Innate immunity in the lungs
Martin, T. R. and Frevert, C. W. (2005), 'Innate immunity in the lungs', *Proc Am Thorac Soc*, 2 (5), 403–11.

Immunity and the skin
Pasparakis, M., Haase, I., and Nestle, F. O. (2014), 'Mechanisms regulating skin immunity and inflammation', *Nat Rev Immunol*, 14 (5), 289–301.

Syndrome X (where a child didn't age)
Walker, R. F., et al. (2009), 'A case study of "disorganized development" and its possible relevance to genetic determinants of aging', *Mech Ageing Dev*, 130 (5), 350–6.

Endorphins
Stefano, G. B., et al. (2012), 'Endogenous morphine: up-to-date review 2011', *Folia Biol (Praha)*, 58 (2), 49–56.

Chapter 2

Winston Churchill quote
Churchill, W. and Langworth, R.M. (2008), *Churchill By Himself: the Life, Times and Opinions of Winston Churchill in His Own Words* (London: Ebury).

Study provides some indirect evidence that marijuana might benefit patients suffering from depression
Korem, N. and Akirav, I. (2014), 'Cannabinoids prevent the effects of a footshock followed by situational reminders on emotional processing', Neuropsychopharmacology, 39 (12), 2709–22.

Even if a bit of marijuana can improve depression, too much seems to make it worse
Bambico, F. R., et al. (2007), 'Cannabinoids elicit antidepressant-like behavior and activate serotonergic neurons through the medial prefrontal cortex', *J Neurosci*, 27 (43), 11700–11.

Systematic review shows that marijuana worsens depressive symptoms
Lev-Ran, S., et al. (2014), 'The association between cannabis use and depression: a systematic review and meta-analysis of longitudinal studies', *Psychol* Med, 44 (4), 797–810.

Book by a group claiming there is a link between vaccines and autism
Conroy, H. (2013), *TheThinking Moms' Revolution: Autism Beyond the Spectrum: Inspiring True Stories From Parents Fighting to Rescue Their Children* (New York, NY: Skyhorse Publishing).

Ben Goldacre's book about things being complicated
Goldacre, B. (2015), *I Think You'll Find It's a Bit More Complicated Than That* (London: Fourth Estate).

Explanations of randomisation, blinding and systematic reviews
Evans, I., Thornton, H., and Chalmers, I. (2010), *Testing Treatments: Better Research for Better Healthcare* (London: Pinter & Martin).
Goldacre, B. (2012), *Bad Pharma: How Drug Companies Mislead Doctors and Harm Patients* (London: Fourth Estate).
Howick, J. (2011), *The Philosophy of Evidence-Based Medicine* (Oxford: Wiley-Blackwell).

Cyclist gets caught with hidden motor
Anonymous (2016), 'A professional cyclist just got caught with an electric motor in her bicycle frame', http://www.techinsider.io/bike-investigated-technological-fraud-cycling-world-championships-cyclocross-2016-1

Pygmalion in the classroom experiment
Rosenthal, R. and Jacobson, L. F. (1992), *Pygmalion in The Classroom: Teacher Expectation and Pupils' Intellectual Development* (New York: Irvington Publishers) p.266.

Pygmalion effects in medicine and management
Learman, L. A., et al. (1990), 'Pygmalion in the nursing home. The effects of caregiver expectations on patient outcomes', *J Am Geriatr Soc*, 38 (7), 797–803.
McNatt, D. B. (2000), 'Ancient pygmalion joins contemporary management: a meta-analysis of the result', *J Appl Psychol*, 85 (2), 314–22.

Evidence that randomisation is often subverted
Schulz, K. F. (1995), 'Subverting randomization in controlled trials', JAMA, 274 (18), 1456–8.

The Oxford – Cambridge Boatrace tie
Anonymous (2014), 'Honest John and the Boat Race legacy', *The Telegraph*.

Vitamin C can reduce the duration of colds in some people
Hemila, H. and Chalker, E. (2013), 'Vitamin C for preventing and treating the common cold', *Cochrane Database Syst Rev*, (1), CD000980.

Ben Goldacre quote: what doctors don't know about the drugs they prescribe (transcript from his TED talk)
TED (2012), 'What doctors don't know about the drugs they prescribe'. http://www.ted.com/talks/ben_goldacre_what_doctors_don_t_know_about_the_drugs_they_prescribe/transcript?language=en

Great article explaining that most trials are never published, and the ones that are published are often hijacked by special interests

Ioannidis, J. P. (2016), 'Evidence-based medicine has been hijacked: a report to David Sackett', *J Clin Epidemiol*.

Article about the crisis within evidence-based medicine due to publication bias (and other problems)

Greenhalgh, T., et al. (2014), 'Evidence based medicine: a movement in crisis?', *BMJ*, 348, g3725.

Hidden biases that favour new drugs almost 100% of the time

Gøtzsche, P. (1989), 'Methodology and overt and hidden bias in reports of 196 double-blind trials of nonsteroidal antiinflammatory drugs in rheumatoid arthritis', *Control Clin Trials*, 10 (1), 31–56.

Why olanzapine beats risperidone, risperidone beats quetiapine, and quetiapine beats olanzapine

Heres, S., et al. (2006), 'Why olanzapine beats risperidone, risperidone beats quetiapine, and quetiapine beats olanzapine: an exploratory analysis of head-to-head comparison studies of second-generation antipsychotics', *Am J Psychiatry*, 163 (2), 185–94.

Study of scientific fraud (industry aren't the only ones who are guilty)

Fanelli, D. (2009), 'How many scientists fabricate and falsify research? A systematic review and meta-analysis of survey data', *PloS one*, 29 May; 4 (5); e5738 (PubMed PMID: 19478950. PubMed Central PMCID: 2685008.)

Systematic review showing that when industry pays for the trial, it is more likely to show that their drug works than if the study is conducted by independent researchers

Bero, L. (2013), 'Industry sponsorship and research outcome: a Cochrane review', *JAMA Intern Med*, 173 (7), 580–1.

The EUROPA study example where a small relative risk reduction was used as evidence that everyone with coronary heart disease should take perindopril, and two books taking apart the claim that small effects matter

Fox, K. M., et al. (2003) (European trial on reduction of cardiac events with perindopril in stable coronary artery disease), 'Efficacy of perindopril in reduction of cardiovascular events among patients with stable coronary artery disease: randomised, double-blind, placebo-controlled, multicentre trial (the EUROPA study)', *Lancet*, 362 (9386), 782–8.

Penston, J. (2010), *Stats. Con – How We've Been Fooled by Statistics-Based Research In Medicine* (London: London Press).

Penston, J. (2003), *Fact And Fiction In Medicalrresearch: The Large-Scale Randomised Trial* (London: London Press).

Cochrane review of the effects of statins, showing they have a clear but small absolute benefit compared with placebo and mild side effects
Taylor, F., et al. (2013), 'Statins for the primary prevention of cardiovascular disease', *Cochrane Database Syst Rev*, 1, CD004816.

Trial showing small benefits of statins for intermediate risk of cardiovascular disease
Yusuf, S., et al. (2016), 'Cholesterol lowering in intermediate-risk persons without cardiovascular disease', *N Engl J Med*, 374 (21), 2021–31.

Trial showing very small benefit of statins for people with a low risk of cardiovascular disease
Zomer, E., et al. (2012), 'Statins for people at low risk of cardiovascular disease', *Lancet*, 380 (9856), 1817; author reply 17–8.

Evidence that exercise is as good as drugs for preventing heart disease, coronary heart disease, rehabilitation after stroke, treatment of heart failure, and prevention of diabetes
Naci, H. and Ioannidis, J. P. (2015), 'Comparative effectiveness of exercise and drug interventions on mortality outcomes: metaepidemiological study', *Br J Sports* Med, 49 (21), 1414–22.

'Expert' review of the evidence for statins (many of the authors have conflicts of interest)
Collins, R., Reith, C., Emberson, J., Armitage, J., Baigent C and Blackwell, L., et al. (2016) 'Interpretation of the evidence for the efficacy and safety of statin therapy', *Lancet*, 19 November; 388 (10059), 2532–61. (PubMed PMID: 27616593.)

Alleged benefits of relative-effect sizes
Barratt, A., et al. (2004), 'Tips for learners of evidence-based medicine:

1. Relative risk reduction, absolute risk reduction and number needed to treat', CMAJ, 171 (4), 353–8.

Back to sleep campaign to prevent sudden infant death syndrome (a good tiny effect)
Gilbert, Ruth, et al. (2005), 'Infant sleeping position and the sudden infant death syndrome: systematic review of observational studies and historical review of recommendations from 1940 to 2002', *IJ Epidemiology*, 34 (4), 874–87.

Discussing putting statins in tap water
Zaman, M. J. and Jones, M. M. (2010), 'Strategies to screen and reduce vascular risk – putting statins in the tap water is not the answer', *Heart*, 96 (3), 177–8.

Spoof recommendation to use parachutes to prevent death
Smith, G. C. and Pell, J. P. (2003), 'Parachute use to prevent death and major trauma related to gravitational challenge: systematic review of randomised controlled trials', *BMJ*, 327 (7429), 1459–61.

Systematic review showing that new treatments are almost as likely to be worse than old treatments as they are to be better
Djulbegovic, B., et al. (2012), 'New treatments compared to established treatments in randomized trials', *Cochrane Database Syst Rev*, 10, MR000024.

The AllTrials campaign is fighting against publication bias, and is making progress
http://www.alltrials.net/

Donald Gillies moped example ('I am different')
Gillies, D. (2000), *Philosophical Theories of Probability* (London: Routledge).

My geeky papers about mechanism
Howick, J., (2011), 'Exposing the vanities – and a qualified defence – of mechanistic evidence in clinical decision-making. *Phil of Sci*, 78 (5); 926–40.
Howick, J., Glasziou, P. and Aronson, J.K., (2010), 'Evidence-based

mechanistic reasoning. *J Royal Soc Med*, November; 103 (11); 433–41. (PubMed PMID: 21037334.)

Howick, J., Glasziou, P., and Aronson, J.K., (2013), 'Problems with using mechanisms to solve the problem of extrapolation', *Theoret Med and Bioethics,* August; 34 (4); 275–91. (PubMed PMID: 23860640. PubMed Central PMCID: 3722444.)

European Carotid Surgery Trial (ECST)
Anonymous (1998), 'Randomised trial of endarterectomy for recently symptomatic carotid stenosis: final results of the MRC European Carotid Surgery Trial (ECST)', *Lancet*, 351 (9113), 1379–87.

Up to 90% of potentially eligible patients are excluded from trials
Mant, D., (1999), 'Can randomised trials inform clinical decisions about individual patients?', *Lancet*, 353 (9154), 743–6.

Penston, J., (2003), *Fact and Fiction In Medical Research: The Large-Scale Randomised Trial* (London: London Press).

Penston, J., (2010), *Stats.Con – How We've Been Fooled By Statistics-Based Research In Medicine* (London: London Press).

Zetin, M. and Hoepner, C.T., (2007), 'Relevance of exclusion criteria in antidepressant clinical trials: a replication study', *J Clin Psychopharmacol*, 27 (3), 295–301.

Zimmerman, M., Mattia, J.I., and Posternak, M.A., (2002), 'Are subjects in pharmacological treatment trials of depression representative of patients in routine clinical practice?', *Am J Psychiatry*, 159 (3), 469–73.

Zimmerman, M., Posternak, M.A., and Chelminski, I. (2002), 'Symptom severity and exclusion from antidepressant efficacy trials', *J Clin Psychopharmacol*, 22 (6), 610–4.

Children respond differently to antidepressants than adults
Bylund, D.B., and Reed, A.L. (2007), 'Childhood and adolescent depression: why do children and adults respond differently to antidepressant drugs?', *Neurochem Int*, 51 (5), 246-53.

Deupree, J.D., Reed, A.L., and Bylund, D.B. (2007), 'Differential effects of the tricyclic antidepressant desipramine on the density of adrenergic receptors in juvenile and adult rats', *J Pharmacol Exp Ther*, 321 (2), 770–6.

Evaluation of the Tamil Nadu Integrated Nutrition Projects (worked in Tamil Nadu but not in Bangladesh because the environment and culture were different

Karim, R., et al. (2003), *The Bangladesh Integrated Nutrition Project: Endline Evaluation Of The Community Based Nutrition Component* (Boston, Dhaka: The Institute of Nutrition and Food Sciences, The Friedman School of Nutrition Science).

Save the Children Federation (2003), *Thin on the Ground. Questioning the Evidence Behind World Bank-funded Community Nutrition Projects in Bangladesh*, (London: Save the Children Federation).

World Bank (1998), *Implementation Completion Report. India. Second Tamil Nadu Integrated Nutrition Project*, (Washington: World Bank, Operations Evaluation Department).

White, Howard (2009), *Theory-Based Impact Evaluation: Principles and Practice', in International Initiative for Impact Evaluation*, (New Delhi: International Initiative for Impact Evaluation).

Chapter 3

Ernst Schumacher quote

Schumacher, E. F. (1993), *Small Is Beautiful : A Study Of Economics As If People Mattered* (London: Vintage).

Mark Twain quote

Beard, D.C. and Stein, B.L. (2011), *A Connecticut Yankee In King Arthur's Court* (Berkeley, CA: University of California Press).

Semmelweis story

Gillies, D. (2005), 'Hempelian and Kuhnian approaches in the philosophy of medicine: the Semmelweis case', *Stud Hist Philos Biol Biomed Sci*, 36 (1), 159–81.

Semmelweis, I. (ed. Carter Codell, K.) (1983), *The Etiology, Concept, and Prophlaxis Of Childbed Fever* (Madison; WI: University of Wisconsin Press).

The anti-arrhythmic drug case

Epstein, A. E., et al. (1993), 'Mortality following ventricular arrhythmia suppression by encainide, flecainide, and moricizine after myocardial infarction. The original design concept of the Cardiac Arrhythmia Suppression Trial (CAST)', *JAMA*, 270 (20), 2451–5.

NIH (1986), 'The cardiac arrhythmia suppression trial (CAST)', in *National Heart, Lung and Blood Institute* (NHLBI) (National Institutes of Health).

Evidence that most people don't want to take drugs with tiny absolute effect sizes

Fontana, M., et al. (2014), 'Patient-accessible tool for shared decision making in cardiovascular primary prevention: balancing longevity benefits against medication disutility', *Circulation*, 129 (24), 2539–46.

The GOBSAT ('Good Old Boys Sat Around a Table') method described

Greenhalgh, T. (2006) How To Read A Paper : The Basics Of Evidence-Based Medicine. 3rd edn (Malden, Mass.: BMJ Books/Blackwell Pub).

Paper about consensus statements to rule whether treatments work (before the dawn of EBM)

Goodman, C. and Baratz, S.R. (1990), *Consensus Development at the NIH: Improving the Program*, ed. Institute of Medicine (Washington, DC: National Academy Press).

Iain Chalmers' story about listing to experts and theory about antibiotics for measles

Chalmers, I. (2002), 'Why we need to know whether prophylactic antibiotics can reduce measles-related morbidity', *Pediatrics*, 109 (2), 312–5.

American Psychiatric Association members have strong link with industry

Cosgrove, L. and Krimsky, S. (2012), 'A comparison of DSM-IV and DSM-5 panel members' financial associations with industry: a pernicious problem persists', *PLOS Med*, 9 (3), e1001190.

Other industries also have conflicts of interest (psychiatry is not alone)

Catala-Lopez, F., Sanfelix-Gimeno, G., Ridao, M. and Peiro, S. (2013) 'When are statins cost-effective in cardiovascular prevention? A systematic review of sponsorship bias and conclusions in economic evaluations of statins', *PLOS One*, 8 (7); e69462. (PubMed PMID: 23861972. Pubmed Central PMCID: 3704635.)

Lexchin, J., Bero, L.A., Djulbegovic, B. and Clark, O. (2003) 'Pharmaceutical industry sponsorship and research outcome and quality: systematic review', *BMJ*, 31 May; 326 (7400); 1167–70. (PubMed PMID: 12775614. Pubmed Central PMCID: 156458. Epub 2003/05/31. eng.)

Study showing that textbooks (written by experts) do not reflect latest evidence and therefore continue to recommend treatments that are useless or harmful

Antman, E. M., et al. (1992), 'A comparison of results of meta-analyses of randomized control trials and recommendations of clinical experts. Treatments for myocardial infarction', *JAMA*, 268 (2), 240–8.

Systematic review of health benefits of fasting (positive but weak evidence)

Horne, B.D., Muhlestein, J.B. and Anderson, J.L. (2015) 'Health effects of intermittent fasting: hormesis or harm? A systematic review.' *Am J Cllin* Nutrit, August; 102 (2), 464–70. (PubMed PMID: 26135345.)

Systematic review of pomegranate for lowering blood pressure and other things

Sahebkar, A., Ferri, C., Giorgini, P., Bo, S., Nachtigal, P. and Grassi, D. (2017) 'Effects of pomegranate juice on blood pressure: A systematic review and meta-analysis of randomized controlled trials.' *Pharmacol Res* January; 115, 149–61. (PubMed PMID: 27888156.)

NHS Choices review of pomegranate evidence: http://www.nhs.uk/Livewell/superfoods/Pages/is-pomegranate-a-superfood.aspx

Systematic review of positive psychology interventions (including the 'Best Possible Self' exercise)

Bolier, L., Haverman, M., Westerhof, G.J., Riper, H., Smit, F., Bohlmeijer, E. (2013) 'Positive psychology interventions: a meta-analysis of randomized controlled studies.' BMC Public Health, 13, 119. (PubMed PMID: 23390882. PubMed Central PMCID: 3599475.)

Chapter 4

Henry Knowles Beecher's systematic review of placebo effects

Beecher, H.K. (1955) 'The powerful placebo', *J Am Med Assoc*, 159 (17); 1602–6.

Beecher, H.K. (1961) 'Surgery as placebo. A quantitative study of bias', *JAMA*, 176; 1102–7.

Article questioning Beecher's method (the 'post hoc ergo procter hoc' fallacy)

Kienle, G.S and Kiene, H. (1997) 'The powerful placebo effect: fact or fiction?', *J Clin Epidemiol*, 50 (12); 1311–8.

Peter Gøtzsche and Asbjorn Hróbjartsson's systematic review comparing placebo with no treatment

Hróbjartsson, A. and Gøtzsche, P. (2001) 'Is the placebo powerless? An analysis of clinical trials comparing placebo with no treatment', *N Engl J Med*, 344 (21); 1594–602.

Hróbjartsson, A. and Gøtzsche, P. (2004) 'Is the placebo powerless? Update of a systematic review with 52 new randomized trials comparing placebo with no treatment', *J Internal Med*, 256 (2); 91–100.

Hróbjartsson, A. and Gøtzsche, P. (2010) 'Placebo interventions for all clinical conditions', *Cochrane Database of Systematic Reviews*, (1); CD003974.

Irving Kirsch noting the problem of heterogeneity in the placebo systematic review

Kirsch, I. (2002) 'Yes, there is a placebo effect, but is there a powerful antidepressant effect?', *Prevention and Treatment*, 5 (22).

My study comparing average treatment effects with average placebo effects

Howick, J., Friedemann, C., Tsakok, M., et al. (2013) 'Are treatments more effective than placebos? A systematic review and meta-analysis', *PlOS One*, 8 (5); e62599.

Studies of Hawthorne effects

De Amici, D., Klersy, C., Ramajoli, F., Brustia, L. and Politi, P. (2000)

'Impact of the Hawthorne effect in a longitudinal clinical study: the case of anesthesia', *Control Clin Trials*, 21 (2); 103–14.

Hanson, D.L. (1967) 'Influence of the Hawthorne effect upon physical education research', *Res Q*, 38 (4); 723–4.

Kohli, E., Ptak, J., Smith, R., Taylor, E., Talbot, E.A and Kirkland, K.B. (2009) 'Variability in the Hawthorne effect with regard to hand hygiene performance in high- and low-performing inpatient care units', *Infect Control Hosp Epidemiol*, 30 (3); 222–5.

Systematic review showing that patients in the 'no treatment' groups within Hróbjartsson and Gøtzsche's placebo systematic review got better

Krogsboll, L.T., Hrobjartsson, A. and Gotzsche, P.C. (2009)' Spontaneous improvement in randomised clinical trials: meta-analysis of three-armed trials comparing no treatment, placebo and active intervention' *BMC Med Res Methodol*, 9; 1.

Systematic review showing that SSRI antidepressants only have tiny effects for depression compared with placebo

Kirsch, I., Deacon, B.J., Huedo-Medina, T.B., Scoboria, A., Moore, T.J. and Johnson, B.T. (2008) 'Initial severity and antidepressant benefits: a meta-analysis of data submitted to the Food and Drug Administration', *PLOS Med*, 5 (2); e45.

Systematic review showing that 'active' placebos are more effective than standard placebos

Moncrieff, J., Wessely, S. and Hardy, R. (2004) 'Active placebos versus antidepressants for depression', *Cochrane Database of Syst Rev*, 1; CD003012.

Trials of 'open label' placebos

Kaptchuk, T.J., Friedlander, E., Kelley, J.M., et al. (2010) 'Placebos without deception: a randomized controlled trial in irritable bowel syndrome', *PlOS One*, 5 (12); e15591.

Sandler, A.D. and Bodfish, J.W. (2008) 'Open-label use of placebos in the treatment of ADHD: a pilot study', *Child Care Health Dev*, 34 (1); 104–10.

Kelley, J.M., Kaptchuk, T., Cusin, C., Lipkin, S. and Fava, M. (2012) 'Open-label placebo for major depressive disorder: A pilot randomized controlled trial', *Psychother and Psychosom*, 81; 312–14.

Ethics of placebos

Howick, J. (2009) 'Questioning the methodologic superiority of "placebo" over "active" controlled trials', *Am J Bioethics*, 9 (9); 34–48.

Foddy, B. (2009) 'A duty to deceive: placebos in clinical practice', *Am J Bioethics*, 9 (12); 4–12.

Interview with Linda Buonanno who said open label placebos made her feel better than ever

Placebos Helping IBS, Migraine Sufferers Find Relief (2016). http://www.youtube.com/watch?v=poYw35TR_SU (accessed 21 September).

Part II
Chapter 5

Rice powder used as a lie detector test in ancient times
Kleinmuntz, B. and Szucko, J. J. (1984), 'Lie detection in ancient and modern times. A call for contemporary scientific study', *Am Psychol*, 39 (7), 766–76.

Walter Cannon and the discovery of the fight or flight response
Cannon, W.B. (1929), *Bodily Changes In Pain, Hunger, Fear and Rage: An Account Of Recent Researches Into The Function Of Emotional Excitement* (2nd edn: College Park).
(1932), *The Wisdom of the Body* (Kegan Paul & Co.: printed in the U.S.A.), pp. xv, 312.

Evidence that people are too stressed out these days
APA (2013), '2013 Work and Well-Being' survey by the American Psychological Association.
Services, Department of Health and Human (1999), 'Mental Health: A Report of the Surgeon General', in US Public Health Service (Pittsburgh, PA).
Taelman, J., et al. (2011), 'Instantaneous changes in heart rate regulation due to mental load in simulated office work', *Eur J Appl Physiol*, 111 (7), 1497–505.

Selye's discovery and description of the stress response
Selye, H. (1976), *The Stress of Life* (rev. edn; New York: McGraw-Hill).

Evidence linking stress with poor health outcomes

Heart disease
Li, J., Zhang, M., Loerbroks, A., Angerer, P., Siegrist, J. (2014) 'Work stress and the risk of recurrent coronary heart disease events: A systematic review and meta-analysis', *Int J Occupational Med and Environmental Health*.

Stress and sleeping disorders

Han, K. S., Kim, L., and Shim, I. (2012), 'Stress and sleep disorder', *Exp Neurobiol*, 21 (4), 141–50.

Depression and heart disease

Meijer, A., et al. (2011), 'Prognostic association of depression following myocardial infarction with mortality and cardiovascular events: a meta-analysis of 25 years of research', *Gen Hosp Psychiatry*, 33 (3), 203–16.

Mahar, I., et al. (2014), 'Stress, serotonin, and hippocampal neurogenesis in relation to depression and antidepressant effects', *Neurosci Biobehav Rev*, 38, 173–92.

Monroe, S. M., Slavich, G. M., and Gotlib, I. H. (2014), 'Life stress and family history for depression: the moderating role of past depressive episodes', *J Psychiatr Res*, 49, 90–5.

Anxiety

Roest, A. M., et al. (2010), 'Prognostic association of anxiety post myocardial infarction with mortality and new cardiac events: a meta-analysis', *Psychosom Med*, 72 (6), 563–9.

Financial stress

Georgiades, A., et al. (2009), 'Financial strain predicts recurrent events among women with coronary artery disease', *Int J Cardiol*, 135 (2), 175–83.

Autoimmune diseases

Temajo, N. O. and Howard, N. (2014), 'The mosaic of environment involvement in autoimmunity: The abrogation of viral latency by stress, a non-infectious environmental agent, is an intrinsic prerequisite prelude before viruses can rank as infectious environmental agents that trigger autoimmune diseases', *Autoimmun Rev*, 13 (6), 635–40.

Angina Pectoris

King, M. S., Carr, T., and D'Cruz, C. (2002), 'Transcendental meditation, hypertension and heart disease', *Aust Fam Physician*, 31 (2), 164–8.

Anxiety and restlessness
Shannahoff-Khalsa, D. S., et al. (1999), 'Randomized controlled trial of yogic meditation techniques for patients with obsessive-compulsive disorder', *CNS Spectr*, 4 (12), 34–47.

Asthma
Rietveld, S., Everaerd, W., and Creer, T. L. (2000), 'Stress-induced asthma: a review of research and potential mechanisms', *Clin Exp Allergy*, 30 (8), 1058-66.
Trueba, A. F. and Ritz, T. (2013), 'Stress, asthma, and respiratory infections: pathways involving airway immunology and microbial endocrinology', *Brain Behav Immun*, 29, 11–27.

Cardiac arrhythmias
Ditto, B., Eclache, M., and Goldman, N. (2006), 'Short-term autonomic and cardiovascular effects of mindfulness body scan meditation', *Ann Behav Med*, 32 (3), 227–34.

Consipation
Vadiraja, S. H., et al. (2009), 'Effects of yoga on symptom management in breast cancer patients: A randomized controlled trial', *Int J Yoga*, 2 (2), 73–9.

Diabetes mellitus
Miller, C. K., et al. (2014), 'Comparison of a mindful eating intervention to a diabetes self-management intervention among adults with type 2 diabetes: a randomized controlled trial', *Health Educ Behav*, 41 (2), 145–54.

Mild and moderate depression
Goyal, M., et al. (2014), 'Meditation programs for psychological stress and well-being: a systematic review and meta-analysis', *JAMA Intern Med*, 174 (3), 357–68.

Fatigue and energy levels
Kim, Y. H., et al. (2013), 'Effects of meditation on anxiety, depression, fatigue, and quality of life of women undergoing radiation therapy for breast cancer', *Complement Ther Med*, 21 (4), 379–87.

Focus

Chan, D. and Woollacott, M. (2007), 'Effects of level of meditation experience on attentional focus: is the efficiency of executive or orientation networks improved?', *J Altern Complement Med*, 13 (6), 651–7.

Kozasa, E. H., et al. (2012), 'Meditation training increases brain efficiency in an attention task', *Neuroimage*, 59 (1), 745–9.

Herpes simplex (cold sores)

Cruess, S., et al. (2000), 'Reductions in herpes simplex virus type 2 antibody titers after cognitive behavioral stress management and relationships with neuroendocrine function, relaxation skills, and social support in HIV-positive men', *Psychosom Med*, 62 (6), 828–37.

Hypertension (high blood pressure)

Barnes, V. A. and Orme-Johnson, D. W. (2006), 'Clinical and pre-clinical applications of the transcendental meditation program in the prevention and treatment of essential hypertension and cardiovascular disease in youth and adults', *Curr Hypertens Rev*, 2 (3), 207–18.

Benson, H., et al. (1974), 'Decreased blood pressure in borderline hypertensive subjects who practiced meditation', *J Chronic Dis*, 27 (3), 163–9.

Immune system

Cohen, S., et al. (1998), 'Types of stressors that increase susceptibility to the common cold in healthy adults', *Health Psychol*, 17 (3), 214–23.

Infertility

Domar, A. D., Seibel, M. M., and Benson, H. (1990), 'The mind/body program for infertility: a new behavioral treatment approach for women with infertility', *Fertil Steril*, 53 (2), 246–9.

Insomnia

Kaul, P., et al. (2010), 'Meditation acutely improves psychomotor vigilance, and may decrease sleep need', *Behav Brain Funct*, 6, 47. http://onlinelibrary.wiley.com/doi/10.1348/135910704773891005/abstract

Pain

Schaffer, S. D. and Yucha, C. B. (2004), 'Relaxation & pain management: the relaxation response can play a role in managing chronic and acute pain', *Am J Nurs*, 104 (8), 75-6, 78-9, 81-2.

Zeidan, F., et al. (2010), 'The effects of brief mindfulness meditation training on experimentally induced pain', *J Pain*, 11 (3), 199–209. http://www.ncbi.nlm.nih.gov/pubmed/23436504

Post-traumatic stress disorder

Chung, M. C. and Wall, N. (2013), 'Alexithymia and posttraumatic stress disorder following asthma attack', *Psychiatr Q*, 84 (3), 287–302.

Rees, B., et al. (2013), 'Reduction in posttraumatic stress symptoms in Congolese refugees practicing transcendental meditation', *J Trauma Stress*, 26 (2), 295–8.

Sexual dysfunction

Hedon, F. (2003), 'Anxiety and erectile dysfunction: a global approach to ED enhances results and quality of life', *Int J Impot Res*, 15 Suppl 2, S16–9.

Substance abuse

Sinha, R., et al. (2000), 'Psychological stress, drug-related cues and cocaine craving', *Psychopharmacology (Berl)*, 152 (2), 140–8.

Teeth problems

Goyal, S., et al. (2013), 'Stress and periodontal disease: the link and logic!!', *Ind Psychiatry J*, 22 (1), 4–11.

Wound healing

Gouin, J. P. and Kiecolt-Glaser, J. K. (2011), 'The impact of psychological stress on wound healing: methods and mechanisms', *Immunol Allergy Clin North Am*, 31 (1), 81–93.

Heart disease leading cause of death worldwide, and it is growing

World Health Organization (2014), 'The top 10 causes of death'.

We have 50 stress responses per day on average (estimate)

Benson, H. (2001), *The Relaxation Response* (HarperCollins).

McEwen, B.S. and Lasley, E.N. (2002), *The End Of Stress As We*

Know It (Washington, DC: Joseph Henry; [Oxford: Oxford Publicity Partnership] [distributor]).

Work stress questionnaire
Sanne, B., et al. (2005), 'The Swedish Demand-Control-Support Questionnaire (DCSQ): factor structure, item analyses, and internal consistency in a large population', *Scand J Public Health*, 33 (3), 166–74.

Mindfulness reduces heart disease
Schneider, R. H., et al. (2012), 'Stress reduction in the secondary prevention of cardiovascular disease: randomized, controlled trial of transcendental meditation and health education in Blacks', *Circ Cardiovasc Qual Outcomes*, 5 (6), 750–8.

Researchers identified 293 studies that showed an impact of stress on the immune system
Segerstrom, S. C. and Miller, G. E. (2004), 'Psychological stress and the human immune system: a meta-analytic study of 30 years of inquiry', *Psychol Bull*, 130 (4), 601–30.

Dhabhar, F. S. (2014), 'Effects of stress on immune function: the good, the bad, and the beautiful', *Immunol Res*, 58 (2-3), 193–210.

Overview with examples of how stress changes physiology
Nakata, A. (2012), 'Psychosocial job stress and immunity: a systematic review', *Methods Mol Biol*, 934, 39–75.

Mechanism linking stress and brain activity
Calcia, M. A., et al. (2016), 'Stress and neuroinflammation: a systematic review of the effects of stress on microglia and the implications for mental illness', *Psychopharmacology (Berl)*, 233 (9), 1637–50.

Alice Herz-Sommer's story (Holocaust survivor who dies at 110 and remained positive her whole life)
Fox, Margalit (2014), 'Alice Herz-Sommer, who found peace in Chopin amid Holocaust, dies at 110', *New York Times*.

Story of Chinese farmer
Chu, Chin-Ning (1991), *The Asian Mind Game: Unlocking The Hidden Agenda Of The Asian Business Culture: A Westerner's Survival*

Manual (New York: Rawson Associates; Oxford: Maxwell Macmillan International).

Chapter 6

Mary Schmich article about chewing bubble gum to solve algebra problems
Schmich, M. (1997), 'Wear sunscreen', *Chicago Tribune*.

Paul McCartney saying 'We'd been into drugs, the next step is, you've got to try and find a meaning then'
Swanson, D. 'The History of the Beatles and the Maharishi', http://ultimateclassicrock.com/the-beatles-india-maharishi/?trackback=tsmclip%3E, accessed.

The relaxation response and how it changes your biology: Benson's initial experiments
Benson, H. (2001), *The Relaxation Response* (Harper Collins).

Relaxing jaw can relax entire body
Mohammadi Fakhar, F., Rafii, F., and Jamshidi Orak, R. (2013), 'The effect of jaw relaxation on pain anxiety during burn dressings: randomised clinical trial', *Burns*, 39 (1), 61–7.

List of different types of meditation
IAM (2014), '8 Basic Kinds of Meditation', <http://www.iam-u.org/index.php/8-basic-kinds-of-meditation-and-why-you-should-meditate-on-your-heart%3E, accessed 11 February 2014.

Systematic reviews of the relaxation response (including 'Bensonian' relaxation, meditation, and yoga) for lowering blood pressure and preventing heart disease
Cramer, H., et al. (2014), 'A systematic review and meta-analysis of yoga for hypertension', *Am J Hypertens*, 27 (9), 1146–51.
Hagins, M., et al. (2013), 'Effectiveness of yoga for hypertension: systematic review and meta-analysis', *Evid Based Complement Alternat Med*, 2013, 649836.
Hartley, L., et al. (2014), 'Transcendental meditation for the primary

prevention of cardiovascular disease', *Cochrane Database Syst Rev*, (12), CD010359.

Hartley, L., et al. (2014), 'Yoga for the primary prevention of cardio-vascular disease', *Cochrane Database Syst Rev*, (5), CD010072.

Nagele, E., et al. (2014), 'Clinical effectiveness of stress-reduction techniques in patients with hypertension: systematic review and meta-analysis', *J Hypertens*, 32 (10), 1936–44; discussion 44.

Rainforth, M. V., et al. (2007), 'Stress reduction programs in patients with elevated blood pressure: a systematic review and meta-analysis', *Curr Hypertens Rep*, 9 (6), 520–8.

More evidence that meditation lowers blood pressure and is recommended by the American Heart Association

Brook, R. D., et al. (2013), 'Beyond medications and diet: alternative approaches to lowering blood pressure: a scientific statement from the american heart association', *Hypertension*, 61 (6), 1360–83.

Gregoski, M. J., et al. (2012), 'Differential impact of stress reduction programs upon ambulatory blood pressure among african american adolescents: influences of endothelin-1 gene and chronic stress exposure', *Int J Hypertens*, 510291.

Kabat-Zinn and the relationship between Buddhist meditation and mindfulness

Ludwig, D. S. and Kabat-Zinn, J. (2008), 'Mindfulness in medicine', *JAMA*, 300 (11), 1350–2.

Systematic review evidence that the relaxation response etc. improves health

Transcendental meditation for preventing heart disease

Hartley, L., et al. (2014a), 'Transcendental meditation for the primary prevention of cardiovascular disease', *Cochrane Database Syst Rev*, 12, CD010359.

Mindfulness reduces depression and anxiety and depression

Goyal, M., et al. (2014), 'Meditation programs for psychological stress and well-being: a systematic review and meta-analysis', *JAMA Intern Med*, 174 (3), 357–68.

Relaxation response and various disorders (systematic review evidence)

Anxiety: reducing anxiety
Kirkwood, G., et al. (2005), 'Yoga for anxiety: a systematic review of the research evidence', *Br J Sports Med*, 39 (12), 884–91; discussion 91.

Arthritis
A systematic review including 11 randomised trials showed a benefit of mindfulness therapy for treating chronic pain (including arthritis):
Bawa, F.L., Mercer, S.W., Atherton, R.J. et al. (2015) 'Does mindfulness improve outcomes in patients with chronic pain? Systematic review and meta-analysis', *B Journal GP*, 65 (635); e387–400.

Low back pain
Cramer, H., et al. (2014), 'A systematic review and meta-analysis of yoga for hypertension', *Am J Hypertens*, 27 (9), 1146–51.

Binge eating: decreases binge eating
Katterman, S.N., Kleinman, B.M., Hood, M.M., Nackers, L.M., Corsica, J.A. (2014) 'Mindfulness meditation as an intervention for binge eating, emotional eating, and weight loss: a systematic review', *Eating Behaviors*, 15 (2): 197–204.

Cancer: improving psychological health of cancer patients
Cramer, H., et al. (2012), 'Yoga for breast cancer patients and survivors: a systematic review and meta-analysis', *BMC Cancer*, 12, 412.

Cognitive decline: offset cognitive decline
Gard, T., Holzel, B. K., and Lazar, S. W. (2014), 'The potential effects of meditation on age-related cognitive decline: a systematic review', *Ann N Y Acad Sci*, 1307, 89–103.

Depression
Klainin-Yobas, P., et al. (2015), 'Effects of relaxation interventions on depression and anxiety among older adults: a systematic review', *Aging Ment Health*, 19 (12), 1043–55.
Piet, J. and Hougaard, E. (2011), 'The effect of mindfulness-based cognitive therapy for prevention of relapse in recurrent major depres-

sive disorder: a systematic review and meta-analysis', *Clin Psychol Rev*, 31 (6), 1032–40.

Diabetes mellitus
Aljasir, B., Bryson, M., and Al-Shehri, B. (2010), 'Yoga practice for the management of type ii diabetes mellitus in adults: a systematic review', *Evid Based Complement Alternat Med*, 7 (4), 399–408.

Innes, K. E. and Vincent, H. K. (2007), 'The influence of yoga-based programs on risk profiles in adults with type 2 diabetes mellitus: a systematic review', *Evid Based Complement Alternat Med*, 4 (4), 469–86.

Hypertension
Bai, Z., et al. (2015), 'Investigating the effect of transcendental meditation on blood pressure: a systematic review and meta-analysis', *J Hum Hypertens*.

Cramer, H., et al. (2014), 'A systematic review and meta-analysis of yoga for hypertension', *Am J Hypertens*, 27 (9), 1146–51.

Rainforth, M. V., et al. (2007), 'Stress reduction programs in patients with elevated blood pressure: a systematic review and meta-analysis', *Curr Hypertens Rep*, 9 (6), 520–8.

Tyagi, A. and Cohen, M. (2014), 'Yoga and hypertension: a systematic review', *Altern Ther Health Med*, 20 (2), 32–59.

Wang, J., Xiong, X., and Liu, W. (2013), 'Yoga for essential hypertension: a systematic review', *PLOS One*, 8 (10), e76357.

Insomnia
Kim, S. M., Park, J. M., and Seo, H. J. (2016), 'Effects of mindfulness-based stress reduction for adults with sleep disturbance: a protocol for an update of a systematic review and meta-analysis', *Syst Rev*, 5, 51.

Neuendorf, R., et al. (2015), 'The effects of mind-body interventions on sleep quality: a systematic review', *Evid Based Complement Alternat Med*, 902708.

Ischaemic heart disease: recovery and secondary prevention for ischaemic heart disease
van Dixhoorn, J. and White, A. (2005), 'Relaxation therapy for rehabilitation and prevention in ischaemic heart disease: a systematic review and meta-analysis', *Eur J Cardiovasc Prev Rehabil*, 12 (3), 193–202.

Irritable bowel syndrome

A systematic review with eight trials suggests that relaxation meditation can reduce IBS symptoms. Park, S-H., Han, K.S. and Kang, C-B. (2014) 'Relaxation therapy for irritable bowel syndrome: a systematic review', *Asian Nursing Research*, 8 (3); 182–92.

Multiple sclerosis (MS): managing MS

Levin, A.B., Hadgkiss, E.J., Weiland, T.J. and Jelinek, G.A. (2014) 'Meditation as an adjunct to the management of multiple sclerosis' *Neuro Res Int*, 704691.

Senders, A., Wahbeh, H., Spain, R. and Shinto, L. (2012) 'Mind-body medicine for multiple sclerosis: a systematic review', *Autoimmune Diseases*, 567324.

Pain: reducing pain

Carroll, D. and Seers, K. (1998) 'Relaxation for the relief of chronic pain: a systematic review', *J Advanced Nursing*, 27 (3); 476–87.

Sheinfeld Gorin, S., Krebs, P., Badr, H., et al. (2012) 'Meta-analysis of psychosocial interventions to reduce pain in patients with cancer', *J Clin Oncology*, 30 (5); 539–47.

Post-traumatic stress disorders

Bisson, J.I., Roberts, N.P., Andrew, M., Cooper, R. and Lewis, C. (2013) 'Psychological therapies for chronic post-traumatic stress disorder (PTSD) in adults', *Cochrane Database Syst Rev*, 12, CD003388.

Pregnancy: positive effects on neonatal outcomes

Fink, N.S., Urech, C., Cavelti, M. and Alder, J. (2012) 'Relaxation during pregnancy: what are the benefits for mother, fetus, and the newborn? A systematic review of the literature.', *J Perinatal and Neonatal Nursing*, 26 (4); 296–306.

Schizophrenia: reducing anxiety in schizophrenic patients

Vancampfort, D., Correll, C.U., Scheewe, T.W., et al. (2013) 'Progressive muscle relaxation in persons with schizophrenia: a systematic review of randomized controlled trials', *Clin Rehab*, 27 (4); 291–8.

Stress: reducing stress

Chong, C.S., Tsunaka, M., Tsang, H.W., Chan, E.P. and Cheung, W.M. (2011) 'Effects of yoga on stress management in healthy adults: A systematic review', *Alternat The Health and Med*, 17 (1); 32–8.

Lower-quality (not from systematic reviews) evidence concerning relaxation response and various disorders (evidence from lower quality studies)

Asthma

Huntley, A., White, A.R. and Ernst, E. (2002) 'Relaxation therapies for asthma: a systematic review', *Thorax*, 57 (2); 127–31.

Pbert, L., Madison, J.M., Druker, S., et al. (2102) 'Effect of mindfulness training on asthma quality of life and lung function: a randomised controlled trial', *Thorax*, 67 (9); 769–76.

Nickel, C., Lahmann, C., Muehlbacher, M., et al. (2006) 'Pregnant women with bronchial asthma benefit from progressive muscle relaxation: a randomized, prospective, controlled trial', *Psychotherapy and Psychosom*, 75 (4); 237–43.

Yorke, J., Fleming, S.L. and Shuldham, C. (2007) 'Psychological interventions for adults with asthma: a systematic review', *Respiratory Med*, 101 (1); 1–14.

Increases wellbeing / happiness

Chang, B.H., Boehmer, U., Zhao, Y. and Sommers, E. (2007) 'The combined effect of relaxation response and acupuncture on quality of life in patients with HIV: a pilot study', *J Alternat and Complement Med*, 13 (8); 807–15.

Kim, Y.H., Kim, H.J., Ahn, S.D., Seo, Y.J. and Kim, S.H. (2013) 'Effects of meditation on anxiety, depression, fatigue, and quality of life of women undergoing radiation therapy for breast cancer', *Complement Ther in Med*, 21 (4); 379–87.

Reduces irritability

Speca, M., Carlson, L.E., Goodey, E. and Angen, M. (2000) 'A randomized, wait-list controlled clinical trial: the effect of a mindfulness meditation-based stress reduction program on mood and symptoms of stress in cancer outpatients', *Psychosom Med*, 62 (5); 613–22.

Drug or alcohol abuse

Haaga, D.A., Grosswald, S., Gaylord-King, C., et al. (2011) 'Effects of the transcendental meditation program on substance use among university students', *Cardiol Res Pract*, 537101.

Shafil, M., Lavely, R. and Jaffe, R. (1975) 'Meditation and the prevention of alcohol abuse', *Am J Psychiatry*, 132 (9); 942–5.

Improves memory

Deffenbacher, K.A., Bornstein, B.H., Penrod, S.D. and McGorty, E.K. (2004) 'A meta-analytic review of the effects of high stress on eyewitness memory', *Law Hum Behav*, 28 (6); 687–706.

Guglietti, C.L., Daskalakis, Z.J., Radhu, N., Fitzgerald, P.B. and Ritvo, P. 'Meditation-related increases in GABAB modulated cortical inhibition', *Brain Stimul*, 6 (3); 397–402.

Study showing the effect of stress on gene expression (see Chapter Fifteen for more references)

Dusek, J.A., Otu, H.H., Wohlhueter, A.L., et al. (2008) 'Genomic counter-stress changes induced by the relaxation response', *PlOS One*, 3 (7); e2576.

The modified candle problem –Glucksberg's original study

Glucksberg, S. (1962) 'The influence of strength of drive on functional fixedness and perceptual recognition', *J Experimental Psychology*, 63, 36–41.

Meditation activates the parasympathetic nervous response

Wu, S.D. and Lo, P.C. (2008) 'Inward-attention meditation increases parasympathetic activity: a study based on heart rate variability', *Biomed Res*, October 29 (5);245–50. (PubMed PMID: 18997439.)

Svenson et al. have written about more research exploring the relationship between stress and (reduced) creativity

Svenson, O. and Maule, A.J. (1993) 'Time pressure and stress in human judgement and decision making', *Plenum*.

Abiola Keller's study showing that worrying about stress is worse than the actual stress

Keller, A., Litzelman, K., Wisk, L.E., et al. (2012) 'Does the perception that stress affects health matter? The association with health and mortality', *Health Psychol*, 31 (5); 677–84.

Relaxation improves the immune system function
Black, D.S. and Slavich, G.M. (2016) 'Mindfulness meditation and the immune system: a systematic review of randomized controlled trials', *Ann New York Acad Sciences*, 1373 (1); 13–24.

The belief that stress is okay reduces the effects of stress
Keller, A., Litzelman, K., Wisk, L.E., et al. (2012) 'Does the perception that stress affects health matter? The association with health and mortality', *Health Psychol*, 31 (5); 677–84.

Eustress and the zone (The Yerkes/Dodson Law)
Yerkes, R.M. and Dodson, J.D. (1908) 'The relation of strength of stimulus to rapidity of habit-formation', *J Comparative Neurology and Psychology*, 18; 459–82.

The sigh of relief
Vlemincx, E., Taelman, J., Van Diest, I., Van den Bergh, O. (2010) 'Take a deep breath: the relief effect of spontaneous and instructed sighs', *Physiol Behav*, 101 (1); 67–73.

Benson's relaxation exercise
Benson, H. (2001) *The Relaxation Response*, New York, HarperCollins.

Williams, M. and Penman, D. (2011)
Mindfulness: A Practical Guide to Finding Peace in a Frantic World, London, Piatkus.

Chapter 7

Bruce Moseley's trial of placebo knee surgery
Moseley, J.B., O'Malley, K., Petersen, N.J., et al. (2002) 'A controlled trial of arthroscopic surgery for osteoarthritis of the knee', *N Eng J Med*, 347 (2); 81–8.

Prevalence of knee arthroscopic surgery

American Orthopaedic Society for Sports Medicine. Knee Arthroscopy. 2015. http://orthoinfo.aaos.org/topic.cfm?topic=a00299 (accessed 26 May 2015).

Kim, S., Bosque, J., Meehan, J.P., Jamali, A. and Marder, R. (2011) 'Increase in outpatient knee arthroscopy in the United States: a comparison of National Surveys of Ambulatory Surgery, 1996 and 2006', *J Bone and Joint Surgery* (American volume), 93 (11); 994–1000.

Placebo controlled vertebroplasty procedure

Buchbinder, R., Osborne, R.H., Ebeling, P.R., et al. (2009) 'A randomized trial of vertebroplasty for painful osteoporotic vertebral fractures', *New Eng J Med*, 361 (6) 557–68.

Staples, M.P., Kallmes, D.F., Comstock, B.A., et al. (2011) 'Effectiveness of vertebroplasty using individual patient data from two randomised placebo controlled trials: meta-analysis' *BMJ*, 343, d3952.

Vertebroplasty prevalence

Long, S.S., Morrison, W.B. and Parker, L. (2012) 'Vertebroplasty and kyphoplasty in the United States: provider distribution and guidance method, 2001-2010', *Am J Roentgenology*, 199 (6); 1358–64.

Vertebropasty can lead to the side-effect of cement leakage

Teng, M.M., Cheng, H., Ho, D.M. and Chang, C.Y. (2006) 'Intraspinal leakage of bone cement after vertebroplasty: a report of 3 cases', *Am J Neuroradiology*, 27 (1); 224–9.

Vertebropasty can increase the risk of adjacent fractures

Lin, E.P., Ekholm, S., Hiwatashi, A. and Westesson, P.L. (2004) 'Vertebroplasty: cement leakage into the disc increases the risk of new fracture of adjacent vertebral body', *Am J Neuroradiology*, 25 (2); 175–80.

Physical therapy can reduce knee pain

Wang, S.Y., Olson-Kellogg, B., Shamliyan, T.A., Choi, J.Y., Ramakrishnan, R. and Kane, R.L. (2012) 'Physical therapy interventions for knee pain secondary to osteoarthritis: a systematic review', *Annals Internal Med, 157 (9)*; 632–44.

Placebo surgery systematic review
Wartolowska, K., Judge, A, Collins, G., et al. (2014) 'Use of placebo controls in the evaluation of surgery: systematic review', *BMJ*, 348, g3253.

Wound healing mechanism
Krafts, K.P. (2010) 'Tissue repair: The hidden drama', *Organogenesis*, 6 (4); 225–33.
Enoch, S and Price, P. (2004) *World Wide Wounds*. http://www.worldwidewounds.com/2004/august/Enoch/Pathophysiology-Of-Healing.html (accessed 7 June 2015).

Exercise for back pain
Hayden, J.A., van Tulder, M.W., Malmivaara, A. and Koes, B.W. (2005) 'Exercise therapy for treatment of non-specific low back pain', *Cochrane Database Systematic Reviews*, 3, CD000335.

Yoga for back pain
Cramer, H., Lauche, R., Haller, H. and Dobos, G. (2013) 'A systematic review and meta-analysis of yoga for low back pain', *Clinical J Pain*, 9 (5); 450–60.

Descartes
Descartes, R, Clarke, D.M. (2011) *Meditations and Other Metaphysical Writings* (London: Folio Society).

Ryle on why Descartes is wrong
Ryle, G. (2009) *The Concept of Mind*. (60th anniversary edn.) (Abingdon: Routledge).

The link between mental and physical illness
Novick, D., Montgomery, W., Kadziola, Z., et al. (2013) 'Do concomitant pain symptoms in patients with major depression affect quality of life even when taking into account baseline depression severity?', *Patient Prefer Adherence*, 7, 463–70.
Trivedi, M.H. (2004) 'The link between depression and physical symptoms', *Primary Care Companion to Journal Clin Psychiatry*, 6 (Suppl 1); 12–6.

The TGN1412 tragic case gone wrong

Goldacre, B. (2012) *Bad Pharma: How Drug Companies Mislead Doctors and Harm Patients.* (London: Fourth Estate).

Coghlan, A. (2006) 'Mystery over drug trial debacle deepens', *New Scientist.*

Suntharalingam, G., Perry, M.R., Ward, S., et al. (2006) 'Cytokine storm in a phase 1 trial of the anti-CD28 monoclonal antibody TGN1412', *New Eng J Med*, 355 (10); 1018–28.

Link between depression and physical symptoms (like pain)

Trivedi. M.H. (2004) 'The link between depression and physical symptoms', *Primary Care Companion to J Clin Psychiatry*, 6 (Suppl 1); 12–6.

Studies on the problems of inferring that something works based on a mechanism picture

Howick, J., Glasziou, P. and Aronson, J.K. (2010) 'Evidence-based mechanistic reasoning', *J Royal Society Med*, 103 (11); 433–41.

Howick, J., Glasziou, P. and Aronson, J.K. (2013) 'Problems with using mechanisms to solve the problem of extrapolation', *Theoretic Med and Bioethics*, 34 (4); 275–91.

Composition of the human body

Emsley, J. (1998) *The Elements.* (3rd edn.; Oxford: Clarendon Press).

Description of the problem of consciousness

van Gulick, R. (2014) 'Consciousness', in: Zalta, E.N. (ed.) *Stanford Encyclopedia of Philosophy.* (Stanford, CA: Metaphysics Research Lab).

Evidence that people in comas are still conscious to some degree

Rosenberg, R.N. (2009)'Consciousness, coma, and brain death', *JAMA*, 301 (11); 1172–4.

Discussion of emergent properties

O'Connor, T. (2015) 'Emergent Properties', in: Zalta, E.N. (ed.) *Stanford Encyclopedia of Philosophy.* (Stanford, CA: Metaphysics Research Lab).

Harrington (which contains Morris quote about Earl Grey Tea)
Harrington, A. (ed.) (1997) *The Placebo Effect: An Interdisciplinary Exploration.*, (Cambridge, MA: Harvard University Press).

Moerman (reply to Earl Grey tea quote)
Moerman, D.E. 'Meaningful placebos – controlling the uncontrollable', *New Engl J Med*, 365 (2); 171–2.

Conservative treatment is as good as surgery for back problems
Zaina, F., Tomkins-Lane, C., Carragee, E. and Negrini, S. (2016) 'Surgical versus non-surgical treatment for lumbar spinal stenosis', *Cochrane Database Syst Rev*, January 29 (1); CD010264. (PubMed PMID: 26824399.)
van Middelkoop, M., Rubinstein, S.M., Kuijpers, T., Verhagen, A.P., Ostelo, R, Koes, B.W., et al. (2011) 'A systematic review on the effectiveness of physical and rehabilitation interventions for chronic non-specific low back pain', *Eur Spine J*, Jan 20 (1); 19–39. (PubMed PMID: 20640863. Pubmed Central PMCID: 3036018.)

... and neck problems
van Middelkoop, M., Rubinstein, S.M., Ostelo, R., van Tulder, M.W., Peul, W., Koes, B.W., et al. (2013) 'Surgery versus conservative care for neck pain: a systematic review', *Eur Spine J*, Jan 22 (1); 87–95. (PubMed PMID: 23104514. Pubmed Central PMCID: 3540296.)

... and hip fractures
Handoll, H.H. and Parker, M.J. (2008) 'Conservative versus operative treatment for hip fractures in adults', *Cochrane Database Syst Rev*, Jul, 16 (3); CD000337. (PubMed PMID: 18646065.)

... and knee problems
Katz, J.N. and Losina, E. (2013) 'Surgery versus physical therapy for meniscal tear and osteoarthritis', *N Engl J Med*, 15 Aug, 369 (7); 677–8. (PubMed PMID: 23944314.)

Part III
Chapter 8

Low doses of amphetamines have an effect on ADHD

Sandler, A.D. and Bodfish, J.W. (2008) 'Open-label use of placebos in the treatment of ADHD: a pilot study', *Child Care Health Dev*, 34 (1); 104–10.

Bruce Thomas study on the power of being positive

Thomas, K.B. (1987) 'General practice consultations: is there any point in being positive?', *BMJ*, 294 (6581); 1200–2.

Benedetti's open versus hidden design (and information about how placebos can induce the body to produce endorphins)

Benedetti, F. (2009) *Placebo Effects : Understanding The Mechanisms In Health and Disease*, (Oxford: Oxford University Press).

My systematic review showing that empathy and positive expectations can reduce symptoms of pain and some other ailments

Howick, J., Fanshawe, T.R., Mebius, A., Lewith, G., Heneghan, C.J., Bishop, F., Little, P., Mistiaen, P. and Roberts, N.W. (2015) 'Effects of changing practitioner empathy and patient expectations in healthcare consultations', *Cochrane Database Syst Rev*, Issue 11, Art. No: CD011934. DOI: 10.1002/14651858.CD011934

Placebos work by reducing anxiety

Petrovic, P., Dietrich, T., Fransson, P., Andersson, J., Carlsson, K. and Ingvar, M. (2005) 'Placebo in emotional processing--induced expectations of anxiety relief activate a generalized modulatory network', *Neuron*, 46 (6); 957–69.

Expectations reduce anxiety (and subsequently reduce pain and depression)

Wager, T.D. (2005) 'Expectations and anxiety as mediators of placebo effects in pain', *Pain*, 115 (3); 225–6.

Staats, P.S., Staats, A. and Hekmat, H. (2001) 'The additive impact of anxiety and a placebo on pain', *Pain* Med, 2 (4); 267–79.

Dopamine, expectations, and pain

Wood, L., Egger, M., Gluud, L.L., et al. (2008) 'Empirical evidence of bias in treatment effect estimates in controlled trials with different interventions and outcomes: meta-epidemiological study', *BMJ*, 336 (7644); 601–5.

Colloca, L. and Benedetti, F. (2007) 'Nocebo hyperalgesia: how anxiety is turned into pain', *Current Opinion in Anaesthesiology*, 20 (5); 435–9.

ADHD sales growth

IMS Institute. (2012) *The Use of Medicines in the United States: Review of 2011*) (Parsippany, NJ: IMS Institute for Healthcare Informatics).

Open versus hidden for Parkinson's and Anxiety and Pain

Benedetti, F. (2009) Placebo Effects: Understanding The Mechanisms In Health and Disease. (Oxford: Oxford University Press).

Placebos and back pain

Linde, K., Witt, C.M., Streng, A., et al.' The impact of patient expectations on outcomes in four randomized controlled trials of acupuncture in patients with chronic pain', *Pain*, 128 (3); 264–71.

Exercise and diet prevent diabetes

Bain, E., Crane, M., Tieu, J., Han, S., Crowther, C.A. and Middleton, P. (2015) 'Diet and exercise interventions for preventing gestational diabetes mellitus', *Cochrane Database SystRev*, 4: CD010443.

Self-efficacy and expectancy (the belief that you can do what it takes to achieve your goals)

Bandura, A. (1997) *Self-Efficacy : The Exercise Of Control* (New York: W.H. Freeman).

Pygmalion studies

Learman, L.A., Avorn, J., Everitt, D.E. and Rosenthal, R. (1990) 'Pygmalion in the nursing home. The effects of caregiver expectations on patient outcomes', *J Am Geriatr Soc*, 38 (7); 797–803.

McNatt, D.B.(2000) 'Ancient pygmalion joins contemporary management: a meta-analysis of the result', *J Appl Psychol*, 85 (2); 314–22.

Rosenthal, R. and Jacobson, L.F. (1998) *Pygmalion In The Classroom:*

Teacher Expectation And Pupils' Intellectual Development, (New York: Irvington Publishers).

Studies showing a link between what the doctor says ('this may hurt') and what the patient feels
Krauss, B.S. (2015) '"This may hurt": predictions in procedural disclosure may do harm', *BMJ*, 350; h649.
Cohen, L.L., MacLaren, J.E., Fortson, B.L., et al. 'Randomized clinical trial of distraction for infant immunization pain', *Pain*, 125 (1-2); 165–71.
Taddio, A., Appleton, M., Bortolussi, R., et al. (2010) 'Reducing the pain of childhood vaccination: an evidence-based clinical practice guideline (summary)', *CMAJ*, 182 (18); 1989–95.

Chinese study of negative words on morphine use
Wang, F., Shen, X., Xu, S., et al. (2008) 'Negative words on surgical wards result in therapeutic failure of patient-controlled analgesia and further release of cortisol after abdominal surgeries', *Minerva Anestesiologica*, 74 (7-8); 353–65.

Nocebo effects - parent distractions
Cohen, L.L., MacLaren, J.E., Fortson, B.L., et al. 'Randomized clinical trial of distraction for infant immunization pain', *Pain*, 125 (1-2); 165–71.

Adverse events in placebo groups within clinical trials of migraine, pain, and epilepsy drugs
Zaccara, G., Giovannelli, F. and Schmidt, D. (2015) 'Placebo and nocebo responses in drug trials of epilepsy', *Epilepsy and Behavior*, 43, 128–34.
Hauser, W., Sarzi-Puttini, P., Tolle, T.R. and Wolfe, F. (2012) 'Placebo and nocebo responses in randomised controlled trials of drugs applying for approval for fibromyalgia syndrome treatment: systematic review and meta-analysis', *Clin and Experimental Rheumatology*, 30 (6 Suppl 74); 78–87.
Amanzio, M., Corazzini, L.L., Vase, L. and Benedetti, F. (2009) 'A systematic review of adverse events in placebo groups of anti-migraine clinical trials', *Pain*, 146 (3); 261–9.

Raj Ragunathan's description of mental chatter

Raghunathan, R. (2013) 'How Negative is Your "Mental Chatter"?', *Psychology Today*. **Fuck it therapy**
Parkin, J.C. (2007) *F**k It : the Ultimate Spiritual Way* (London: Hay House).

Chapter 9

Weinberg quote
Weinberg, S. (1993) *Dreams Of A Final Theory* (London: Vintage).

The link between mental and physical illness
Novick, D., Montgomery, W., Kadziola, Z., et al. (2013) 'Do concomitant pain symptoms in patients with major depression affect quality of life even when taking into account baseline depression severity?' *Patient Prefer Adherence*,7, 463–70.
Trivedi, M.H. (2004) 'The link between depression and physical symptoms', *Primary Care Companion to J Clin Psychiatry*, 6 (Suppl 1); 12–6.

Open label placebo studies
Park, L.C. and Covi, L. (1965) 'Nonblind Placebo Trial: an Exploration of Neurotic Patients' Responses to Placebo When Its Inert Content Is Disclosed', *Archives Gen Psychiatry*, 12, 36–45.
Petkovic, G., Charlesworth, J.E., Kelley, J., Miller, F., Roberts, N. and, Howick, J. (2015) 'Effects of placebos without deception compared with no treatment: protocol for a systematic review and meta-analysis', *BMJ*, 5 (11); e009428.

Even single cells can be conditioned
Ridge, J.P., Di Rosa, F. and Matzinger, P. (1998) 'A conditioned dendritic cell can be a temporal bridge between a CD4+ T-helper and a T-killer cell', *Nature*, 393 (6684); 474–8.

Pavlovian conditioning
Benedetti, F., Carlino, E. and Pollo, A. (2011) 'How placebos change the patient's brain'. *Neuropsychopharmacology*, 36 (1); 339–54.

Producing allergy with plastic rose

MacKenzie, J.N. (1886) 'The production of the so-called "rose cold" by means of an artificial rose', *Am J Life Sciences*, 91, 45-7.

Ader's description of his studies

Ader, R. (2003) 'Conditioned immunomodulation: research needs and directions', *Brain,Bbehavior, and Immunity*, 17 Suppl 1: S51-7.

Goebel's study of conditioned immunosuppression in humans

Goebel, M.U., Trebst, A.E., Steiner, J., et al. (2002) 'Behavioral conditioning of immunosuppression is possible in humans', *FASEB*, 16 (14); 1869-73.

Colloca replicates Goebel's study

Colloca, L., Petrovic, P., Wager, T.D., Ingvar, M. and Benedetti, F. (2010) 'How the number of learning trials affects placebo and nocebo responses', *Pain*, 151 (2); 430-9.

Debate over difference between expectancy and conditioning

Stewart-Williams, S. and Podd, J. (2004) 'The placebo effect: dissolving the expectancy versus conditioning debate', *Psycholog Bull*, 130 (2); 324-40.

Active dopamine reward systems associated with placebo responses

Benedetti, F. (2009) *Placebo Effects : Understanding The Mechanisms In Health and Disease* (Oxford: Oxford University Press).

Knutson, B. and Cooper, J.C. (2005) 'Functional magnetic resonance imaging of reward prediction', *Current Opinion Neurology*, 18 (4); 411-7.

Most thoughts subconscious

Soon, C.S., Brass, M., Heinze, H.J. and Haynes, J.D. (2008) 'Unconscious determinants of free decisions in the human brain', *Nature Neuroscience*, 11 (5); 543-5.

Part IV

World Health Organization quote about the definition of health
Leppo, N.E. (1958) 'The first ten years of the World Health Organization', *Minnesota Med*, 41 (8); 577–83.

Susan Pinker's Village Effect
Pinker, S.A. (2014) *The Village Effect : Why Face-To-Face Contact Matters* (New York: Speigel & Graw).

Chapter 10

Patrick O'Brian quote
O'Brian, P. (1970) *Master and Commander* (Bath: Chivers Press).

Quesalid story
Levi-Strauss, C. (1968) *Structural Anthropology* (London: Allen Lane).

My systematic review of surveys showing that while some practitioners do demonstrate empathy, many are less good (or don't have enough time)
Howick, J., Steinkopf, L., Ulyte, A., Roberts, A.N. and Meissner, K. (2017) 'How empathetic is your doctor? A systematic review and meta-analysis of patient surveys.' (forthcoming).

Atul Gawande's *Being Mortal*
Gawande, A. (2014) *Being Mortal: Illness, Medicine and What Matters In the End* (London: Profile).

The Aetna insurance company study showing that patients in palliative care live longer
Krakauer, R., Spettell, C.M., Reisman, L. and Wade, M.J. (2009) 'Opportunities to improve the quality of care for advanced illness', *Health Affairs*, 28 (5); 1357–9.

Discussion of other studies that replicate the Aetna study
Parikh, R.B., Kirch, R.A., Smith, T.J. and Temel, J.S. (2013) 'Early

specialty palliative care--translating data in oncology into practice',
New Eng J Med, 369 (24); 2347–51.

Some authors have questioned the link between serotonin and depression

Cowen, P.J. and Browning, M. (2015) 'What has serotonin to do with depression?', *World Psychiatry*, *14 (2); 158–60.*

Systematic reviews showing that practitioner empathy improves patient outcomes

Derksen, F., Bensing, J., Lagro-Janssen, A. (2013) 'Effectiveness of empathy in general practice: a systematic review', *Br J Gen Pract*, 63 (606); e76-84.

Mistiaen, P., van Osch, M., van Vliet, L., et al. (2016) 'The effect of patient-practitioner communication on pain: a systematic review', *Eur J Pain*, 20 (5); 675–88.

Kelley, J.M., et al. (2014) 'The influence of the patient-clinician relationship on healthcare outcomes: A systematic review and meta-analysis of randomized controlled trials', *PLOS One*, 9 (4); e94207.

Kelm, Z., Womer, J., Walter, J.K. and Feudtner, C. (2014) 'Interventions to cultivate physician empathy: a systematic review', *BMC Med Educ*, 14, 219.

Randomised trial showing that training doctors in empathy increases their empathy

Riess, H., Kelley, J.M., Bailey, R.W., Dunn, E.J. and Phillips, M. (2012) 'Empathy training for resident physicians: a randomized controlled trial of a neuroscience-informed curriculum', *J Gen Intern Med*, 27 (10); 1280–6.

Evidence that the immune system can use up a lot of energy

Kominsky, D.J., Campbell, E.L. and Colgan, S.P. (2010) 'Metabolic shifts in immunity and

Inflammation', *J Immunology*, *184(8); 4062–8.*
Segerstrom, S.C.(2007) 'Stress, energy, and immunity: an ecological view', Current Directions in Psycholog Science, 16 (6); 326–30.

Randomised trial of empathy training reduce patient anxiety
Little, P., White, P., Kelly, J., Everitt, H. and Mercer, S.W. (2015) 'Randomised controlled cluster trial of a brief intervention to improve non-verbal communication in general practice consultations', under review.

Randomised trial of an augmented consultation to treat irritable bowel syndrome
Kaptchuk, T.J., Kelley, J.M., Conboy, L.A. et al. (2008) 'Components of placebo effect: randomised controlled trial in patients with irritable bowel syndrome', *BMJ*, 336 (7651); 999–1003.

Animal studies shows there is a cost to launching the full immune response
Demas, G.E., Chefer, V., Talan, M.I. and Nelson, R.J. (1997) 'Metabolic costs of mounting an antigen-stimulated immune response in adult and aged C57BL/6J mice', *Am J Physiol*, 273 (5 Pt 2); R1631–7.

Hanssen, S.A., Hasselquist, D., Folstad, I. and Erikstad, K.E. (2004) 'Costs of immunity: immune responsiveness reduces survival in a vertebrate', *Proc Biol Sciences/The Royal Society*, 271 (1542); 925–30.

Vangronsveld study of negative words and lack of empathy harming patients
Vangronsveld, K.L. and Linton, S.J. (2012) 'The effect of validating and invalidating communication on satisfaction, pain and affect in nurses suffering from low back pain during a semi-structured interview', *Euro J Pain*, 16 (2); 239–46.

Evidence showing that practitioner empathy may also reduce practitioner burnout and improve
Thomas, M.R., Dyrbye, L.N., Huntington, J.L., Lawson, K.L., Novotny, P.J., Sloan, J.A., et al. (2007) 'How do distress and well-being relate to medical student empathy? A multicenter study' *J Gen Internal Med*, Feb 22 (2); 177–83. (PubMed PMID: 17356983. Pubmed Central PMCID: 1824738.)

Kelm, Z,. Womer, J., Walter, J.K. and Feudtner, C. (2014) 'Interventions to cultivate physician empathy: a systematic review', *BMC Med Educ*, 14; 219. (PubMed PMID: 25315848. Pubmed Central PMCID: 4201694.)

DiLalla, L.F., Hull, S.K., Dorsey, J.K., Department of F, Community

Medicine SIUSoMCUSAlse. (2004) 'Effect of gender, age, and relevant course work on attitudes toward empathy, patient spirituality, and physician wellness', *Teaching and Learning in Med*, Spring, 16 (2); 165–70. (PubMed PMID: 15276893.)

Shanafelt, T.D., West, C., Zhao, X., Novotny, P., Kolars, J., Habermann, T, et al. (2005) 'Relationship between increased personal well-being and enhanced empathy among internal medicine residents', *J Gen Internal Med*, July, 20 (7); 559–64. (PubMed PMID: 16050855. PubMed Central PMCID: 1490167.)

Aspirin side-effects

Choices, N. (2016) *Aspirin*. http://www.nhs.uk/conditions/Anti-platelets-aspirin-low-dose-/Pages/Introduction.aspx (accessed 26 November 2016).

Nocebo effects cause dropouts in placebo arms of clinical trials of Parkinsons and other diseases

Stathis, P., Smpiliris, M., Konitsiotis, S. and Mitsikostas, D.D. (2013) 'Nocebo as a potential confounding factor in clinical trials for Parkinson's disease treatment: a meta-analysis', *Eur J Neurol*, 20 (3); 527–33.

Mitsikostas, D.D., Chalarakis, N.G., Mantonakis, L.I., Delicha, E.M. and Sfikakis, P.P. (2012) 'Nocebo in fibromyalgia: meta-analysis of placebo-controlled clinical trials and implications for practice', *Eur J Neurol*, 19 (5); 672–80.

Mitsikostas, D.D., Mantonakis, L.I. and Chalarakis, N.G. (2011) 'Nocebo is the enemy, not placebo. A meta-analysis of reported side effects after placebo treatment in headaches', *Cephalalgia*, 31 (5); 550–61.

The Oxman–Chalmers–Sackett alternative informed consent

Oxman, A.D., Chalmers, I., and Sackett, D.L. (2001) 'A practical guide to informed consent to treatment', *BMJ*, 323 (7327); 1464–6.

Chapter 11

Stories about dying of a broken heart

Hodgekiss, A. (2013) 'You really CAN die of a broken heart: Surviving spouses have a 66% higher risk of dying in the three months after their partner's death', *Daily Mail*, 15 November.

Shakespeare's Tempest

Shakespeare, W. (ed. Kermode, F.) (1988) *The Tempest* (6th edn, London: Routledge).

Chinese Americans who have a birth year combination that is considered ill-fated die younger than non-Chinese Americans

Phillips, D.P., Ruth, T.E. and Wagner, L.M. (1993) 'Psychology and survival', *Lancet*, 342 (8880); 1142–5.

Takotsubo syndrome

Ghadri, J.R., Sarcon, A., Diekmann, J., et al. (2016) 'Happy heart syndrome: role of positive emotional stress in takotsubo syndrome', *Eur Heart J*.

Studies linking widowhood and marriage with life expectancy

Andrade, L., Caraveo-Anduaga, J.J., Berglund, P., et al. (2003) 'The epidemiology of major depressive episodes: results from the International Consortium of Psychiatric Epidemiology (ICPE) Surveys', *Int J Methods in Psychiat Res*, 12 (1); 3–21.

Moon, J.R., Glymour, M.M., Vable, A.M., Liu, S.Y. and Subramanian, S.V. (2014) 'Short- and long-term associations between widowhood and mortality in the United States: longitudinal analyses', *J Public Health*, 36 (3); 382–9.

Shor, E., Roelfs, D.J., Curreli, M., Clemow, L., Burg, M.M. and Schwartz, J.E. (2012) 'Widowhood and mortality: a meta-analysis and meta-regression', *Demography*, 49 (2); 575–606.

Systematic review linking loneliness with mortality (including details of individual studies)

Holt-Lunstad, J., Smith, T.B., Baker, M., Harris, T. and Stephenson, D. (2015) 'Loneliness and social isolation as risk factors for mortality: a meta-analytic review', *Perspectives on Psychological Science*, 10 (2); 227–37.

Marc Schoen's book claiming that because we are too comfortable we activate the fight or flight response for too many silly little things. The book makes sense but is not based on randomised trial evidence.

Shoen, M. (2014) *Your Survival Instinct Is Killing You: Retrain Your Brain to Conquer Fear and Build Resilience*(New York: Plume Books).

Vitamin C does not reduce frequency of colds but reduces the symptom duration once we catch a cold (a systematic review)

Hemila, H. and Chalker, E. (2013) Vitamin C for preventing and treating the common cold', *Cochrane Database Syst* Rev, 1: CD000980.

Association between a spouse dying and mortality

Hodgekiss, A. (2013) 'You really CAN die of a broken heart: Surviving spouses have a 66% higher risk of dying in the three months after their partner's death', *Daily* Mail, 15 November.

Moon, J.R., Glymour, M.M., Vable, A.M., Liu, S.Y. and Subramanian, S.V. (2014) 'Short- and long-term associations between widowhood and mortality in the United States: longitudinal analyses', *J Public Health*, 36 (3); 382–9.

Social networks make us live longer

House, J.S., Landis, K.R. and Umberson, D. (1988) 'Social relationships and health', *Science*, 241 (4865); 540–5.

Holt-Lunstad, J., Smith, T.B. and Layton, J.B. (2010) 'Social relationships and mortality risk: a meta-analytic review' *PLoS Med*, 7 (7); e1000316.

Rosengren, A., Orth-Gomer, K., Wedel, H. and Wilhelmsen, L. (1993) 'Stressful life events, social support, and mortality in men born in 1933', *BMJ*, 307 (6912); 1102–5.

Sheldon Cohen describes his study and the mechanisms by which social networks improve health

Cohen, S. and Janicki-Deverts, D. 'Can We Improve Our Physical Health by Altering Our Social Networks?', *Perspectives on Psycholog Science*.

You are more likely to quit smoking if your friends quit smoking

Christakis, N.A. and Fowler, J.H. (2008) 'The collective dynamics of smoking in a large social network', *New Eng J* Med, 358 (21); 2249–58.

Systematic review of studies showing we are more likely to engage in unhealthy behaviours after a bereavement
Stahl, S.T. and Schulz, R. (2014) 'Changes in routine health behaviors following late-life bereavement: a systematic review', *J Behavioral Med*, 37 (4); 736–55.

Social networks reduces the likelihood of depression after a heart attack
Berkman, L.F., Blumenthal, J., Burg, M., et al. (2003) 'Effects of treating depression and low perceived social support on clinical events after myocardial infarction: the enhancing recovery in coronary heart disease patients (ENRICHD) randomized trial', JAMA, 289 (23); 3106–16.

The widowhood effect
Shor, E., Roelfs, D.J., Curreli, M., Clemow, L., Burg, M.M. and Schwartz, J.E. (2012) 'Widowhood and mortality: a meta-analysis and meta-regression', *Demography*, 49 (2); 575–606.

The stress buffering hypothesis
Cohen, S. and Wills, T.A. (1985) 'Stress, social support, and the buffering hypothesis', *Psycholog* Bull, 98 (2); 310–57.

Oxytocin and social support
Heinrichs, M., Baumgartner, T., Kirschbaum, C. and Ehlert, U. (2003) 'Social support and oxytocin interact to suppress cortisol and subjective responses to psychosocial stress', *BiologPpsychiatry*, 54 (12); 1389–98.
Tom, N. and Assinder, S.J. (2010) 'Oxytocin in health and disease', *Int J Biochem and Cell Biology*, 42 (2); 202–5.

Swedish study of social support protecting against stress
Rosengren, A., Orth-Gomer, K., Wedel, H. and Wilhelmsen, L. (1993) 'Stressful life events, social support, and mortality in men born in 1933', *BMJ*, 307 (6912); 1102–5.

Social support reduces colds
Cohen, S., Frank, E., Doyle, W.J., Skoner, D.P., Rabin, B.S. and Gwaltney, J.M. Jr. (1998) 'Types of stressors that increase susceptibility to the common cold in healthy adults', *Health Psychol*, 17 (3); 214–23.

Experiments on maternal deprivation in humans (these are overviews because there are too many individual studies to cite)
Casler, L. (1961) 'Maternal deprivation: a critical review of the literature', *Monographs of the Soc for Res in Child Development*, 26 (2) 1–64.

Bowlby, J. (1951) 'Maternal care and mental health : a report prepared on behalf of the World Health Organization\2026', (Geneva: WHO).

Spitz, R.A. (1945) 'Hospitalism; an inquiry into the genesis of psychiatric conditions in early childhood', *The Psychoanalytic Study of the Child*, 1, 53–74.

Karen, R. (1994) *Becoming Attached : Unfolding The Mystery Of The Infant-Mother Bond and Its Impact On Later Life.* (New York: Warner).

Experiments on maternal deprivation in monkeys
Kaufman, I.C. and Rosenblum, L.A. (1967) 'The reaction to separation in infant monkeys: anaclitic depression and conservation-withdrawal', *Psychosoma Med*, 29 (6); 648–75.

Kaufman, I.C. and Rosenblum, L.A. (1967) 'Depression in infant monkeys separated from their mothers', *Science*, 155 (3765); 1030–1.

Kaufman, I.C. and Rosenblum, L.A. (1969) 'Effects of separation from mother on the emotional behavior of infant monkeys', *Ann New York Acad Sciences*, 159 (3); 681–95.

Harlow, H.F., Gluck, J.P. and Suomi, S.J. (1972) 'Generalization of behavioral data between nonhuman and human animals.', *Am Psychologist*, 27 (8); 709–16.

Rosenblum, L.A. (1999) 'Experimental studies of susceptibility to panic', project period 2/1/88-8/31/98. NIMH Grant award MH-42545.

Great article about the difference between a real and a 'fake' cause (spurious correlation)
Aschwanden, C. *You Can't Trust What You Read About Nutrition* http://fivethirtyeight.com/features/you-cant-trust-what-you-read-

about-nutrition/?utm_content=buffer9e097&utm_medium=so-
cial&utm_source=twitter.com&utm_campaign=buffer.

Chapter 12

Story about man with Alzheimer's whose heart (but not brain) knew it was Mother's Day
McGlensey, M. (2014) 'Man with Alzheimer's proves that even if the mind forgets, "the heart remembers"', *Huffington Post*.

Hartman, S. (2014) 'As man's mind fades, heart comes to the rescue', *CBS News*.

Randomised trial of health benefits of volunteering
George, D.R. and Singer, M.E. (2011) 'Intergenerational volunteering and quality of life for persons with mild to moderate dementia: results from a 5-month intervention study in the United States', *Am J Geriatr Psychiatry*, 19 (4); 392–6.

Systematic review of health benefits of volunteering
Jenkinson, C.E., Dickens, A.P., Jones, K., et al. (2013) 'Is volunteering a public health intervention? A systematic review and meta-analysis of the health and survival of volunteers', *BMC Public Health*, 13, 773.

Randomised trial showing that volunteering changes the biology of the volunteers
Schreier, H.M., Schonert-Reichl, K.A. and Chen, E. (2013) 'Effect of volunteering on risk factors for cardiovascular disease in adolescents: a randomized controlled trial', *JAMA Pediatrics*, 167 (4); 327–32.

Article about man who jumped in front of a subway to save someone
BBC. (2007) 'NY subway "hero" saves teenager'.

Evolutionary explanation for altruism: the unit of evolution is not our genes
Axelrod, R. and Hamilton, W.D. (1981) 'The evolution of cooperation', *Science*, 211 (4489); 1390–6.

Altruistic motivations for altruistic behaviours improve health more than selfish motivations

Konrath, S., Fuhrel-Forbis, A., Lou, A. and Brown, S. (2012) 'Motives for volunteering are associated with mortality risk in older adults', *Health* Psychol, 31 (1); 87–96.

People who care for family members with dementia develop numerous health problems

Pinquart, M. and Sorensen, S. (2007) 'Correlates of physical health of informal caregivers: a meta-analysis', *J of Gerontology, Series B*, Psychological sciences and social sciences, 62 (2); P126–37.

Oxytocin and social support

Heinrichs, M., Baumgartner, T., Kirschbaum, C. and Ehlert, U. (2003) 'Social support and oxytocin interact to suppress cortisol and subjective responses to psychosocial stress', *Biological Psychiatry*, 54 (12); 1389–98.

Tom, N. and Assinder, S.J. (2010) 'Oxytocin in health and disease', *Int J Biochemistry and Cell Biology*, 42 (2); 202–5.

The benefits of gratitude

Emmons, R.A. and McCullough, M.E. (2003) 'Counting blessings versus burdens: an experimental investigation of gratitude and subjective well-being in daily life', *Journal Personality and Social Psychol*, 84 (2); 377–89.

Eid, M. and Larsen, R.J. (2008) *The Science Of Subjective Well-Being* (New York and London: Guilford).

Mirror neurons

Rizzolatti, G. and Craighero, L. (2004), 'The mirror-neuron system', *Annu Rev Neurosci*, 27, 169–92.

Helping others helps the helper and the person helped

Pagano, M.E., Friend, K.B., Tonigan, J.S. and Stout, R.L. (2004) 'Helping other alcoholics in alcoholics anonymous and drinking outcomes: findings from project MATCH', *J Studies on Alcohol*,65 (6); 766–73.

Schwartz, C.E. (1999) 'Teaching coping skills enhances quality of life more than peer support: results of a randomized trial with multiple sclerosis patients', *Health Psychol*, 18 (3); 211–20.

Spiegel, D., Bloom, J.R., Kraemer, H.C. and Gottheil, E. (1989) 'Effect of psychosocial treatment on survival of patients with metastatic breast cancer', *Lancet*, 2 (8668); 888–91.

Mustafa, M., Carson-Stevens, A., Gillespie, D. and Edwards, A.G. (2013) 'Psychological interventions for women with metastatic breast cancer', *Cochrane Database Syst Rev*, 6, CD004253.

Dale, J., Caramlau, I.O., Lindenmeyer, A. and Williams, S.M. (2008) 'Peer support telephone calls for improving health', *Cochrane Database Syst Rev*, 4, CD006903.

Just thinking about doing good boosts your immune system

McClelland, M. and Nelson, M. (1988) 'The effect of site-specific DNA methylation on restriction endonucleases and DNA modification methyltransferases – a review', *Gene*, 74 (1), 291–304.

And so does giving away money you received as part of an experiment

Moll, J., Krueger, F., Zahn, R., Pardini, M., de Oliveira-Souza, R. and Grafman, J. (2006) 'Human fronto-mesolimbic networks guide decisions about charitable donation', *Proc Nat Acad Sciences of the United States of America*, 103 (42); 15623–8.

Too much volunteering (in the wrong way) can be detrimental to health

Ziersch, A.M. and Baum, F.E. (2004) 'Involvement in civil society groups: Is it good for your health?', *J Epidemiol and Community Health*, 58 (6); 493–500.

Relationship between 'voluntourism' and child trafficking

Punaks, M. and Feit, K. (2014) *The Paradox of Orphanage Volunteering: Combating Child Trafficking Through Ethical Voluntourism*. (Eugene, OR: Next Generation Nepal).

Giving time to volunteer makes you feel like you have more time

Mogilner, C., Chance, Z. and Norton, M.I. (2012) 'Giving time gives you time', *Psycholog Science*, 23 (10); 1233–8.

Part V

Website claims that thoughts can cure diseases:
Mercola, J. (2016) *How Your Thoughts Can Cause or Cure Cancer*
http://articles.mercola.com/sites/articles/archive/2008/02/19/
how-your-thoughts-can-cause-or-cure-cancer.aspx (accessed 28
November).

Website says you can 'think yourself into a new person'
Storr, W. (2014) Can You Think Yourself Into a Different Person?,
Pacific Standard.

Chapter 13

**Angelina Jolie reports that her doctors state she had an 87% chance
of breast cancer (and that people with the BRCA1 gene have a 65%
chance of getting it, on average). She doesn't state how she came up
with the figure of 87%.**
Jolie, A. (2013) 'My medical choice', *New York Times*, 14 May.

**Meta-analysis of studies that investigate the link between BRCA1 genes
and breast cancer (suggests 57%)**
Chen, S. and Parmigiani, G. (2007) 'Meta-analysis of BRCA1 and
BRCA2 penetrance', *J Clin Oncol*, 25 (11); 1329–33.

Watson and Crick's discovery of DNA
Watson, J.D. and Crick, F.H. (1953) 'Molecular structure of nucleic
acids; a structure for deoxyribose nucleic acid', *Nature*, 171 (4356);
737–8.

The exaggerated claims of the Human Genome Project
Rose, H. and Rose, S. (2014) *Genes, Cells and Brains : The Promethean
Promises Of the New Biology* (London: Verso Books).
Hall, S.S. (2010) 'Revolution postponed: why the human genome
project has been disappointing', *Scientific Am.*

Claim that there is a gene for depression
Birkett, J.T., Arranz, M.J., Munro, J., Osbourn, S., Kerwin, R.W. and

Collier, D.A. (2000) 'Association analysis of the 5-HT5A gene in depression, psychosis and antipsychotic response', *Neuroreport*, 11 (9); 2017–20.

Claim that there is a gene for autism
Berkel, S., Marshall, C.R., Weiss, B., et al. (2010) 'Mutations in the SHANK2 synaptic scaffolding gene in autism spectrum disorder and mental retardation', *Nature Genetics*, 42 (6); 489–91.

Claim that there is a gene for happiness
Okbay, A., Baselmans, B.M., De Neve, J.E., et al. (2016) 'Genetic variants associated with subjective well-being, depressive symptoms, and neuroticism identified through genome-wide analyses', *Nature Genetics*, 48 (6); 624–33.

Dr Eric Lander and the failure of the Human Genome Project
Nova Online. Meet the decoders: Dr Eric Lander. 2001. http://www.pbs.org/wgbh/nova/genome/deco_lander.html (accessed 18 May 2015).

Enucleated cells (cells with their nucleus removed) still live
Goldman, R.D., Pollack, R. and Hopkins, N.H. (1973) 'Preservation of normal behavior by enucleated cells in culture', *Pro Nat Acad Sciences of the United States of Am*, 70 (3); 750–4.

The Tabula Rasa theory
Skinner, B. (1976) *About Behaviorism*. (New York: Vintage Books).

Skinner and Watson's radical behaviourism
Schneider, S.M. and Morris E.K. (1987) 'A history of the term radical behaviorism: From Watson to Skinner', *Behavior Analyst*, 10 (1); 27–39.

Charles Darwin & Evolutionary theory
Herbert, S. (2011) *Charles Darwin and The Question Of Evolution: A Brief History With Documents*. (Boston, M.A.: Bedford/St Martin's).

Lamarckism
Gershenowitz, H. (1978) 'The treatment of Lamarckism as found in

forty-one college textbooks', *Indian Journal History of Science*, 13 (2); 144–50.

Deichmann, U. (2016) 'Why epigenetics is not a vindication of Lamarckism - and why that matters', *Studies in History and Philos Biologic and Biomed Sciences*, 57, 80–2.

Evolutionary theory and capitalism

Bergman, J. (2001) 'Darwin's Influence on Ruthless Laissez Faire Capitalism', *Acts & Facts*, 30 (3).

Weisman's claim that Lamarckism is dead

Gauthier, P. (1990) 'Does Weismann's experiment constitute a refutation of the lamarckian hypothesis', *BIOS*, 61 (1/2); 6–8.

The study about people from Överkalix in Sweden who inherited something from their grandparents who had survived a famine

Kaati, G., Bygren, L.O. and Edvinsson, S. (2002) 'Cardiovascular and diabetes mortality determined by nutrition during parents' and grand-parents' slow growth period', *Eur J Human Genetics*, 10 (11); 682–8.

Pembrey, M., Saffery, R. and Bygren, L.O. (2014) 'Network in Epigenetic E. Human transgenerational responses to early-life experience: poten-tial impact on development, health and biomedical research', *J Med Genetics*, 51 (9); 563–72.

Dean Ornish's study of men who changed their diet and lifestyle changed their risk of prostate cancer

Ornish, D., Magbanua, M.J., Weidner, G. et al. (2008) 'Changes in prostate gene expression in men undergoing an intensive nutrition and lifestyle intervention', *Proc Nat Acad Sciences of the United States of America*, 105 (24); 8369–74.

Article about junk DNA

Palazzo, A.F. and Gregory, T.R. (2014) 'The case for junk DNA', *PLOS Genetics*, 10 (5); e1004351.

The potential influence of stress on DNA

Poljsak, B. and Milisav, I. (2012) 'Clinical implications of cellular stress responses', *Bosnian J Basic Med Sciences (Udruzenje basicnih medi-ciniskih znanosti = Association of Basic Medical Sciences)*, 12 (2); 122–6.

Vinkers, C.H., Kalafateli, A.L., Rutten, B.P., et al. (2015) 'Traumatic stress and human DNA methylation: a critical review', *Epigenomics*, 7 (4); 593–608.

Houtepen, L.C., Vinkers, C.H., Carrillo-Roa, T., et al. (2016) 'Genome-wide DNA methylation levels and altered cortisol stress reactivity following childhood trauma in humans', *Nature Communications*, 7; 10967.

Link between BRCA1, BCRA2 and breast cancer

This study suggests that having the BRCA1 gene leads to a 65% risk of breast cancer.

This more recent study suggests it is closer to 57%

Two systematic reviews are beginning to show support for Ornish's conclusions

Deng, W., Cheung, S.T., Tsao, S.W., Wang, X.M. and Tiwari, A.F. (2016) 'Telomerase activity and its association with psychological stress, mental disorders, lifestyle factors and interventions: A systematic review', Psychoneuroendocrinology, 64; 150–63.

Cecile Janssens's study showing that most diseases are about half inherited

Janssens, A.C. and van Duijn, C.M. (2010) 'An epidemiological perspective on the future of direct-to-consumer personal genome testing', *Investigative Genetics*, 1 (1); 10.

Studies claiming that lifestyle accounts for 90% of cancers

Anand, P., Kunnumakkara, A.B., Sundaram, C., et al. (2008) 'Cancer is a preventable disease that requires major lifestyle changes', *Pharmaceutical Res* 25 (9); 2097–116.

Sumamo, E., Ha, C., Korownyk, C., Vandermeer, B. and Dryden, D.M. (2011) *Lifestyle Interventions for Four Conditions: Type 2 Diabetes, Metabolic Syndrome, Breast Cancer, and Prostate* Cancer, (Rockville (MD).

Wu, S., Powers, S., Zhu, W. and Hannun, Y.A. (2016) 'Substantial contribution of extrinsic risk factors to cancer development', *Nature*, 529 (7584); 43–7.

Chapter 14

Theories of personality – where do they come from?
Bynum, W.F.E. and Porter, R. (1993) *Companion Encyclopedia of the History of Medicine. Vol 2* (London: Routledge).

A neural network model of personality types

Berdahl, C.H. (2010) 'A neural network model of Borderline Personality Disorder', *Neural Networks* (the official journal of the International Neural Network Society), 23 (2); 177–88.
Wood, W. and Neal, D.T. (2007) 'A new look at habits and the habit-goal interface' *Psychological Rev*, 114 (4); 843–63.
Gonzalez-Heydrich, J. (1993) 'Using neural networks to model personality development', *Med Hypotheses*, 41 (2); 123–30.
Quek, M. and Moskowitz, D. (2006) 'Testing neural network models of personality' *J Res Personality*, 41 (3); 700–6.

Summary of studies linking genes to personality (the evidence is mixed)
Van Gestel, S. and Van Broeckhoven, C. (2003) 'Genetics of personality: are we making progress?', *Molecular Psychiatry*, 8 (10); 840–52.

Norman Doidge's classic book about neuroplasticity, containing all the stories about Taub and Bach-y-Rita
Doidge, N. (2008) *The Brain That Changes Itself: Stories Of Personal Triumph From the Frontiers Of Brain Science* (London: Penguin Books).

Studies of sensory substitution (using the tongue to see etc.)
Bach-y-Rita, P., Collins, C.C., Saunders, F.A., White, B. and Scadden, L. (1969) 'Vision substitution by tactile image projection', *Nature*, 221 (5184); 963–4.
Bach-y-Rita, P. (2004) 'Tactile sensory substitution studies', *Ann New York Acad Sciences*, 1013; 83–91.

Taub's experiments
Taub, E. and Morris, D.M. (2001) 'Constraint-induced movement therapy to enhance recovery after stroke', *Current Atherosclerosis Reports*, 3 (4); 279–86.

Evidence for constraint-induced movement therapy (CIMT)

Taub, E. and Morris, D.M. (2001) 'Constraint-induced movement therapy to enhance recovery after stroke', *Current Atherosclerosis Reports*, 3 (4); 279–86.

Chen, Y.P., Pope, S., Tyler, D. and Warren, G.L. (2014) 'Effectiveness of constraint-induced movement therapy on upper-extremity function in children with cerebral palsy: a systematic review and meta-analysis of randomized controlled trials', *Clin Rehab*, 28 (10); 939–53.

Fleet, A., Page, S.J., MacKay-Lyons, M. and Boe, S.G. (2014) 'Modified constraint-induced movement therapy for upper extremity recovery post stroke: what is the evidence?', *Topics in Stroke Rehab*, 21 (4); 319–31.

Richards, D. (2008) 'Handsearching still a valuable element of the systematic review', *Evidence-based Dentistry*, 9 (3); 85.

Wolf, S.L., Newton, H., Maddy, D., et al. (2007) 'The Excite Trial: relationship of intensity of constraint induced movement therapy to improvement in the wolf motor function test', *Restorative Neurology and Neuroscience*, 25 (5–6); 549–62.

Medical students' brains change in just months while preparing for exams

Draganski, B., Gaser, C., Kempermann, G., et al. (2006) 'Temporal and spatial dynamics of brain structure changes during extensive learning', *J Neuroscience*, 26 (23); 6314–7.

William James (1890) claims that brains are not hard wired

James, W. (1998) *The Principles of Psychology*. (Bristol: Thoemmes).

Explanation of neuroplasticity in the brain and how it works

Pascual-Leone, A., Freitas, C., Oberman, L., et al. (2011) 'Characterizing brain cortical plasticity and network dynamics across the age-span in health and disease with TMS-EEG and TMS-fMRI', *Brain Topography*, 24 (3-4); 302–15.

Historical (pre-1960) experiments with neuroplasticity

Rosenzweig, M.R. (1996) 'Aspects of the search for neural mechanisms of memory', *Annu Rev Psychology*, 47; 1–32.

Variability hypothesis of evolution (why our brains are plastic)
Potts, R. (1999) 'Variability selection in hominid evolution', *Evolutionary Anthropology*, 7; 81–96.

Most thoughts subconscious
Soon, C.S., Brass, M., Heinze, H.J. and Haynes, J.D. (2008) 'Unconscious determinants of free decisions in the human brain', *Nature Neuroscience*, 11 (5); 543–5.

It takes 2 months to change a habit
Lally, P., van Jaarsveld, C.H., Potts, H.W. and Wardle, J. (2009) 'How are habits formed: Modelling habit formation in the real world', *Eur J Social Psychology*, 40; 998–1009.

The relationship between habits and goals
Wood, W. and Neal, D.T. (2007) 'A new look at habits and the habit-goal interface', *Psycholog Rev*, 114 (4): 843–63.

Review paper explaining the relationship between emotions and the brain; the conclusion is that emotions are better represented as neural networks
Lindquist, K.A., Wager, T.D., Kober, H., Bliss-Moreau, E. and Barrett, L.F. (2012) 'The brain basis of emotion: a meta-analytic review', *Behavioral and Brain Sciences*, 35 (3); 121–43.

Duhigg's book on habits
Duhigg, C. (2012) The Power of Habit : Why We Do What We Do and How To Change. (London: William Heinemann).

Epilogue

My epilogue was inspired by the end of Dan Moerman's wonderful book
Moerman, D.E. (2002) *Meaning, Medicine, and the 'Placebo Effect'*. Cambridge:
Cambridge University Press).